COTA Examination
Review Manual

A Practical Guide to Receiving
Professional Certification

Second Edition

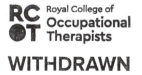

RC◯ Royal College of
◯T Occupational
Therapists

WITHDRAWN

0 0 0 0 2 2 5 8

COTA Examination Review Manual

A Practical Guide to Receiving Professional Certification

Second Edition

M. Teresa Mohler, MA, OTR/L, Ret
Assistant Professor
Mount Aloysius College
Cresson, PA

With

Sherry Pfister, AAS, COTA/L
Academic Fieldwork Coordinator
Mount Aloysius College
Cresson, PA

SLACK Incorporated, 6900 Grove Road, Thorofare, New Jersey 08086-9447

Publisher: John H. Bond
Editorial Director: Amy E. Drummond
Creative Director: Linda Baker
Assistant Editor: Miriam Priest

Printed in the United States of America

Mohler, M. Teresa
     COTA examination review manual: a practical guide to receiving professional certification/M. Teresa Mohler.—2nd ed.
     p. cm.
     Includes bibliographical references and index.
     ISBN 1-55642-346-2 (alk. paper)
     1. Occupational therapy assistants—Examinations, questions, etc.
     2. Occupational therapy—Examinations, questions, etc. I. Title.
     [DNLM: 1. Occupational Therapy—examination questions. 2. Allied Health Personnel—examination questions. WB 18.2 M698c 1997]
RM735.32.M64 1997
615.8'515'076—dc21
DNLM/DLC   97-8104
for Library of Congress

Published by: SLACK Incorporated
                     6900 Grove Road
                     Thorofare, NJ 08086-9447 USA
                     Telephone: 609-848-1000
                     Fax: 609-853-5991

Contact SLACK Incorporated for more information about other books in this field or about the availability of our books from distributors outside the United States.

Last digit is print number: 10 9 8 7 6 5 4 3 2 1

Dedication

This book is dedicated to all occupational therapy assistants
and to Mount Aloysius College graduates in particular
who inspire me and for whom I hold a special place in my heart.

Contents

Dedication v

Acknowledgments ix

Preface xi

Preparation Guidelines xiii

Section I.   **Kinesiologic Concepts**   **1**

Section II.   **Theory**   **17**
    Part A. Pediatrics 19
    Part B. Physical Dysfunction 33
    Part C. Psychosocial Dysfunction 55
    Part D. Media 72

Section III.   **Administration and Management**   **95**

Section IV.   **Occupational Therapy Intervention**   **115**
    Part A. Pediatrics 117
    Part B. Physical Dysfunction 131
    Part C. Psychosocial Dysfunction 156

Section V.   **Ethics and Fieldwork**   **177**

Bibliography 201

Index 205

Acknowledgments

A number of individuals gave invaluable help and advice during the preparation of this book. The author gratefully extends her thanks to the following persons, listed alphabetically:

Janice Bowman, Associate in Specialized Business Secretary, Allied Health Division, Mount Aloysius College, Cresson, PA

E. Nelson Clark, MS, OTR/L Chairman, Allied Health Division, Mount Aloysius College, Cresson, PA

Sister Maria Josephine D'Angelo, RSM, BFA, Professor of Art, Mount Aloysius College, Cresson, PA

Sister Mary Cyrilla Kendra, RSM, BA, Professor of English, Mount Aloysius College, Cresson, PA

Patricia E. Marvin, MA, OTR/L, Private Practice Consultant, Western Pennsylvania

Jacqueline A. Matejovich, Associate Degree in Professional Secretary, Secretary, Allied Health Division, Mount Aloysius College, Cresson, PA

Russell K. Mohler, PT, Chief Physical Therapist, Hollidaysburg Veterans Home, Hollidaysburg, PA

Sister M. Margaretta Phillips, RSM, MA, COTA/L, Associate Professor of Occupational Therapy, Mount Aloysius College, Cresson, PA

Sherry Pfister, AAS, COTA/L, Academic Fieldwork Coordinator, OTA Program, Lecturer, Mount Aloysius College, Cresson, PA

Paul Tryninewski, MPS, PT, Director, Keystone Rehabilitation Systems, Altoona, PA

Bonnie Wareham, OTR/L, Department Head of the Easter Seal Society, Blair and Bedford Counties, Pennsylvania Occupational Therapy Consultant, Rehabilitation Hospital of Altoona, Altoona, PA

Kim Witkovski, OTR/L, Staff Occupational Therapist in Special Interest Section—Psychosocial OT, Altoona Hospital, Altoona, PA

Administrators of Mount Aloysius College, Cresson, PA, who were very supportive of this endeavor.

Preface

Many of my occupational therapy assistant students, as well as new graduates, have sought guidance regarding the preparation for the Certification Examination. This book of questions and answers has been written to provide a review tool to meet those needs. It is an attempt to include comprehensive coverage of occupational therapy theory and intervention.

Best of luck to all of you.

M. Teresa Mohler

Preparation Guidelines for the Certification Exam

Dear graduates of an occupational therapy program:

During your academic life you likely had sufficient experience in studying for tests, and you also acquired a specific learning style. Nevertheless, it is with anxiety, which is considered commonplace, that you await the certification examination. A few practical suggestions will help you manage the exam.

1. Upon conclusion of Fieldwork II your focus is on the exam, and you must know how to handle the stress that is peculiar to this situation. The use of relaxation techniques is a concrete way to face the future with confidence.

   a. Recall the successful moments in your life and allow yourself a "pat on the back."

   b. Use positive reinforcers such as "pep talks" when you reach your goals, motivating you to continue the study process.

   c. Establish support systems among family members and friends, and voice your concerns and feelings for reassurance.

   d. Perform physical exercise every day, such as walking, in combination with deep breathing, which relaxes tense muscles.

   e. Think about activities that are very pleasant to you; e.g., swimming, going on vacation, running, etc.

   f. Follow a healthy and consistent schedule of getting up early in the morning and going to bed early at night.

2. The material that you need to study is primarily from the following sources: the textbooks studied during your school years, the handouts received in this period of time, the notes taken in the classroom, and the cumulative knowledge acquired in community services, Fieldwork I, and Fieldwork II. Do not try to read every piece of material that you collected during the academic years because you will be overwhelmed. Rather, make priority lists based on the "examination content outline for certified occupational therapy assistants" shown here at the end of the guidelines.

3. You must set specific, realistic study goals and attempt to achieve them as closely as you would when recording patient documentation. It will be helpful if you establish a schedule of study to fulfill your objectives: consistency, discipline, and organization are key words to develop good study habits.

4. The National Board of Certification in Occupational Therapy, Inc. (NBCOT) (formerly the American Occupational Therapy Certification Board [AOTCB]) has current information concerning the certification examination review mini courses offered at various

locations, (usually OT schools) throughout the United States. These conferences last 1 to 2 days and are extremely valuable as they focus on the priority areas of the exam. For more information contact the NBCOT directly at:

800 S. Frederick Avenue

Suite 200

Gaithersburg, MD 20877-4150

5. Many applicants find it useful to study for the examination periodically, together with a friend, or in a group, so the knowledge can be exchanged based on the diversified fieldwork experiences of the various members. If you decide to study with others, be sure to choose people with whom you are compatible. Keep in mind that each group must have a leader in order to function efficiently.

6. It is strongly recommended that every applicant receive a good night's sleep before the examination so the mind is clear and refreshed. Do not try to study in the morning when writing the exam. Instead of helping you it will only be confusing.

7. If you feel that you are not sure of the correct answer to a question, do not panic, move on, and come back to it later. Be very careful when changing answers, you must be quite sure when doing so. Do not waste time on subjects that you do not know but try to make the best guess. If you leave the answer blank, it is scored wrong. Read the question without overinterpreting it, and consider the four options carefully before choosing one. Bring several sharpened number 2 pencils with erasers to save time.

8. The certification examination has a total of 200 multiple choice questions, with four options each, to be answered in a 4-hour period. As a result, one must pace oneself in such a way that by the end of the first hour, approximately 50 questions have been answered. It is of the utmost importance to budget one's time in order to be able to complete the exam without hurrying at the end. Running out of time is very disturbing and frustrating. The questions as they appear in the exam are not distributed according to subject materials, they are all mixed together to simulate the patient/client load that you will be treating in actual practice.

9. After the completion of the exam do not worry unnecessarily about the outcome, because you cannot change anything. You did your best and as such should feel good about it.

10. Within 4 to 6 weeks the results will be mailed to you and no one else. On occasion, the candidate must notify his or her employer immediately to address liability problems. You should also contact the support systems, or even consider professional help to cope with the depression that may follow. Do not feel self-conscious about it because most everyone needs this type of help at various times in their lives. In 6 months you can retake the exam, so you must discipline yourself to study and review, the sooner the better. You must analyze yourself to assess what went wrong the first time, and correct those weaknesses. Concentrate on the areas that you know less, rather than the ones you are strong in. The second time around you will know a little more of what to expect and this in itself, is comforting.

11. For your information, the following six pages are the approximate percentages of questions, documented in their entirety by the NBCOT.

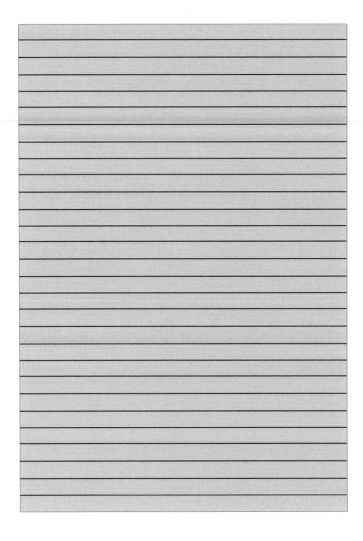

SECTION I

Kinesiologic Concepts

Select the Most Appropriate Answer

1. The word "proximal" means:
   A. Farther from the origin of the body part
   B. Above, toward the head
   C. Closer to the origin of the body part
   D. On the outer side of the body

2. The anatomical frontal or coronal plane is one which:
   A. Divides the body equally into right and left portions
   B. Divides the body equally into front and back portions
   C. Divides the body into superior and inferior portions
   D. Is parallel to the midsagittal plane

3. A multiaxial joint is one of the following:
   A. Ball and socket
   B. Pivot
   C. Ginglymus
   D. Gliding

4. Abduction of the wrist is provided by the:
   A. The palmaris longus
   B. The flexor carpi radialis
   C. The extensor carpi radialis brevis
   D. The extensor carpi radialis longus
   E. B and D
   F. A and C

5. Innervation of the biceps is:
   A. Musculocutaneous
   B. Axillary
   C. Ulnar
   D. Median

6. The tendon of the palmaris longus can be palpated in the anterior area of the wrist:
    A. On the radial side
    B. On the ulnar side
    C. In between A and B
    D. None of the above

7. The function(s) of the lumbricals are:
    A. Flexion of the metacarpophalangeal joints (MCPJs) and proximal interphalangeal joints (PIPJs)
    B. Flexion of the PIPJs and distal interphalangeal joints (DIPJs)
    C. Flexion of the MCPJs and extension of the PIPJs and DIPJs
    D. Flexion of the DIPJs and extension of the MCPJs and DIPJs

8. The wrist extensors are innervated by the:
    A. Radial
    B. Ulnar
    C. Median
    D. Axillary

9. Innervation of the adductor pollicis is:
    A. Median
    B. Radial
    C. Musculocutaneous
    D. Ulnar

10. The flexor pollicis brevis is innervated by the:
    A. Ulnar nerve
    B. Radial nerve
    C. Median and ulnar nerves
    D. Median nerve

11. Key pinch is a prehension pattern in which:
    A. One uses the palmar area of the index finger and thumb tips
    B. One uses the radial area of the index finger and the palmar side of the thumb
    C. One uses the ulnar side of the index finger and the palmar side of the thumb
    D. One uses the radial side of the index finger and the thumb

12. The word supination means:
    A. Turning on an axis
    B. Turning the palm up
    C. Turning the palm down
    D. Turning toward the fifth finger side of the hand

13. The periosteum is:
    A. The lining of the medullary canal
    B. The membrane that covers osseous tissue
    C. The growth plate of the bone
    D. The membrane that covers the external area of the heart

14. When flexion of the elbow is graded "fair," it means that the:
    A. Patient is able to perform the movement antigravity
    B. Patient is able to perform the movement antigravity plus moderate resistance
    C. Patient is unable to perform the movement
    D. Patient is able to perform the movement with gravity eliminated

15. When a person is in standing anatomical position, the wall facing him or her is:
    A. In the transverse plane
    B. In the frontal plane
    C. In the sagittal plane
    D. In the parasagittal plane

16. In standing position, flex the right shoulder and elbow to a 90° angle each, and extend the wrist and fingers pointing to the ceiling, with the forearm in neutral position. In which plane is the right upper extremity located?
    A. The transverse
    B. The frontal
    C. The parasagittal
    D. None of the above

17. In anatomical position, abduct the left shoulder and flex the elbow to a 90° angle each. Extend the wrist and fingers pointing to the front with the palm down. In which plane is the left upper extremity located?
    A. The frontal
    B. The transverse
    C. The sagittal
    D. None of the above

18. How many bones are in a normal adult human hand, excluding the wrist?

    A. 18
    B. 13
    C. 27
    D. 19

19. Which of these movements are performed by the wrist joint?

    A. Flexion and extension
    B. Supination and abduction
    C. Radial and ulnar deviation
    D. Pronation and flexion
    E. A and D
    F. A and C

20. The two main functions of the hand are:

    A. Feeding and pinch
    B. Resting and opposition
    C. Circumduction and grasp
    D. Pinch and grasp

21. Which two muscles in the arm work mainly at the elbow joint?

    A. The levator scapulae and the triceps brachii
    B. The serratus anterior and the biceps brachii
    C. The triceps and the biceps femoris
    D. The biceps brachii and the triceps brachii

22. Which two bones compose the skeleton of the forearm?

    A. The clavicle
    B. The radius
    C. The scapula
    D. The ulna
    E. The tibia
    F. The fibula

23. The three most important motor nerves in the hand are: (select 3 answers)

    A. The ulnar
    B. The sciatic
    C. The radial
    D. The musculocutaneous
    E. The femoral
    F. The abducent
    G. The median

24. The deltoid muscle is divided into three portions; what are they? (select 3 answers)

    A. Superior
    B. Anterior
    C. Posterior
    D. Inferior
    E. Middle
    F. Ventral

25. When one is in standing anatomical position, the ceiling is in the:

    A. Coronal plane
    B. Sagittal plane
    C. Horizontal plane
    D. Vertical plane

26. Which of the prehension patterns does one use when writing?

    A. Key
    B. Fingertip
    C. Palmar tripod
    D. Lateral
    E. Cylindrical

27. A ligament attaches:

    A. Muscle to bone
    B. Muscle to muscle
    C. Bone to bone
    D. Muscle to tendon

28. The brachioradialis is the prime mover on the flexion of the elbow when:
    A. The forearm is in neutral position
    B. The forearm is in complete supination
    C. The forearm is in complete pronation
    D. It does not matter

29. The average measurement of the MCPJ of the second finger is:
    A. 0° to 90°
    B. 0° to 70°
    C. 0° to 60°
    D. 0° to 105°

30. The average measurement of elbow flexion is:
    A. 0° to 90°
    B. 0° to 100°
    C. 0° to 135°
    D. None of the above

31. The hamstrings are muscles that work at the knee and hip joints. They are which of the following?
    A. The tibialis anterior and the biceps femoris
    B. The semitendinosus and the tibialis posterior
    C. The tibialis posterior and the tibialis anterior
    D. The sartorious and the semimembranosus
    E. The biceps femoris
    F. The semimembranosus and the semitendinosus
    G. A and B
    H. E and F

32. Muscles that perform adduction of the fingers are called:
    A. The adductor pollicis
    B. The dorsal interossei
    C. The palmar interossei
    D. The lumbricals

33. The movements that occur at the elbow are:
    A. Supination, flexion, and extension
    B. Flexion and extension
    C. Flexion, extension, and pronation
    D. Pronation and supination

34. Inversion of the ankle is a combination of two other movements; they are:
    A. Supination and adduction
    B. Supination and abduction
    C. Pronation and adduction
    D. Pronation and abduction

35. Which of the following muscles abducts the shoulder?
    A. The posterior deltoid
    B. The serratus anterior
    C. The middle deltoid
    D. The pectoralis major

36. Which of the following is one of the quadriceps?
    A. Semitendinosus
    B. Biceps femoris
    C. Hipstring
    D. Rectus femoris

37. The trapezius is a big muscle of the shoulder girdle that has three portions called:
    A. Anterior, medial, and posterior
    B. Lower, middle, and upper
    C. Anterior, upper, and posterior
    D. Anterior, middle, and posterior

38. The shoulder girdle has movements of its own that occur at the following joints:
    A. Glenohumeral
    B. Sternoclavicular
    C. Acromioclavicular
    D. B and C
    E. A and B

39. Which of the following is *not* a movement performed by the shoulder girdle?
    A. Upward rotation
    B. Internal rotation
    C. Abduction of the scapula
    D. Elevation of the shoulder

40. The lateral movement of the scapula is called:
    A. Retraction
    B. Downward rotation
    C. External rotation
    D. Abduction

41. The coxofemoral joint is a ball and socket, one in which the following movements occur:
    A. Flexion, extension, internal and external rotation, abduction, and adduction
    B. Flexion, extension, abduction, adduction, elevation, and depression
    C. Flexion, extension, upward and downward rotation, abduction, and adduction
    D. Flexion, extension, elevation, depression, abduction, and adduction

42. When the sternocleidomastoideus works bilaterally at the neck it performs:
    A. Lateral flexion
    B. Forward flexion
    C. Extension
    D. Rotation

43. Considering good body mechanics, which of the following provides the greatest amount of stability?
    A. A high center of gravity
    B. A large base of support
    C. A small base of support
    D. All the above

44. The largest peripheral nerve of the body is the:
    A. Radial
    B. Femoral
    C. Sciatic
    D. Musculocutaneous

45. What is commonly known as the "funny bone" of the elbow is actually the:
    A. Ulnar nerve
    B. Median nerve
    C. Radial nerve
    D. Axillary nerve

46. A muscle, which is immobilized in a cast because of a fracture of the bone(s) within the surrounding area, is subject to:

    A. Hyperplasia
    B. Dystrophy
    C. Hypertrophy
    D. Atrophy

47. The dura mater is one of the following membranes of the spinal cord:

    A. Outermost
    B. Innermost
    C. Top to bottom
    D. None of the above

48. The word "nystagmus" means:

    A. Hypersensitive eyes
    B. Burning sensation of the eyes
    C. Nervous twitching of the mouth
    D. Rhythmic oscillation of the eyeballs

49. The strongest tendon of the body is the tendon of the:

    A. Iliopsoas
    B. Gastrocnemius and soleus
    C. Quadriceps
    D. Hamstrings

50. Posteriorly, the scapula has two fossas: the supraspinous and infraspinous, which are separated by the:

    A. Superior border
    B. Acromion
    C. Spine
    D. Inferior angle

51. The pelvic bone is formed by the:

    A. Pubis
    B. Ischium
    C. Patella
    D. Calcaneus
    E. Ilium
    F. A, B, and E

52. The hamstrings are prime movers at the hip and knee; their functions are:
    A. Knee flexion and hip extension
    B. Knee extension and hip flexion
    C. Knee flexion and hip abduction
    D. Knee extension and hip adduction

53. The functions of the biceps brachii and the triceps at the elbow are:
    A. Neutralizers
    B. Agonists
    C. Antagonists
    D. Fixators

54. Muscles that are essentially responsible for the movement of a body part are called:
    A. Synergists
    B. Prime movers
    C. Neutralizers
    D. Antagonists

55. How many muscles does one have in the thumb?
    A. Six
    B. Seven
    C. Eight
    D. Five

56. The median nerve has mainly:
    A. Sensory distribution
    B. Motor distribution
    C. Equal sensory and motor distribution
    D. All the above

57. Which of the following muscles abducts the scapula?
    A. The middle trapezius
    B. The rhomboids
    C. The serratus anterior
    D. The posterior deltoid

58. When the rectus abdominis contracts bilaterally it performs:

    A. Forward flexion
    B. Extension
    C. Rotation of the trunk
    D. Lateral flexion

59. Anatomically speaking, what is the difference between a cavity and a fossa?

    A. A cavity is more convex than a fossa
    B. A cavity is deeper than a fossa
    C. A cavity is shallower than a fossa
    D. A cavity is less concave than a fossa

60. One of the following muscles performs adduction of the scapula:

    A. The upper trapezius
    B. The middle trapezius
    C. The supraspinatus
    D. The subscapularis

61. The location of the neck of the humerus is:

    A. Above the head of the humerus
    B. Below the tubercles
    C. Above the tubercles
    D. Proximal to the tubercles

62. One of these muscles is not attached to the humerus:

    A. The pectoralis minor
    B. The pectoralis major
    C. The triceps
    D. The biceps

63. The following pair of muscles are antagonists, *except*:

    A. Flexor carpi ulnaris versus extensor carpi radialis longus
    B. Biceps versus triceps
    C. Palmaris longus versus flexor carpi radialis
    D. Flexor digitorum profundus versus extensor digitorum

64. The abduction of the scapula is weakened by the loss of the:
    A. Latissimus dorsi
    B. Middle trapezius
    C. Teres major
    D. Serratus anterior

65. Shoulder hyperextension is severely limited by the loss of the:
    A. Middle deltoid
    B. Posterior deltoid
    C. Teres major
    D. Pectoralis major

66. Considering the shoulder joint with the individual in the anatomical position:
    A. Flexion–extention movements take place in a frontal plane
    B. Flexion–extention movements take place in a sagittal plane
    C. Abduction–adduction movements take place in a frontal plane
    D. Abduction–adduction movements take place in a transverse plane

Answer Key

Section I

Kinesiologic Concepts

1. C. Closer to the origin of the body part. **2.** B. Divides the body equally into front and back portions. **3.** A. Ball and socket. **4.** E. Both B) The flexor carpi radialis and D) The extensor carpi radialis longus. **5.** A. Muscolocutaneous. **6.** C. In between A and B. **7.** C. Flexion of the MCPJs and extension of the PIPJs and DIPJs. **8.** A. Radial. **9.** D. Ulnar. **10.** C. Median and ulnar nerves.

11. B. One uses the radial area of the index finger and the palmar side of the thumb. **12.** B. Turning the palm up. **13.** B. The membrane that covers osseous tissue. **14.** A. Patient is able to perform the movement antigravity. **15.** B. In the frontal plane. **16.** C. The parasagittal. **17.** B. The transverse. **18.** D. 19. **19.** F. Both A) Flexion and extension and C) Radial and ulnar deviation. **20.** D. Pinch and grasp.

21. D. The biceps brachii and the triceps brachii. **22.** B) The radius and D) The ulna. **23.** A) The ulnar, C) The radial, and G) The median. **24.** B) Anterior, C) Posterior, and E) Middle. **25.** C. Horizontal plane. **26.** C. Palmar tripod. **27.** C. Bone to bone. **28.** A. The forearm is in neutral position. **29.** A. 0° to 90°. **30.** C. 0° to 135°.

31. H. Both E) The biceps femoris and F) The semimembranosus and semitendinosus. **32.** C. The palmar interossei. **33.** B. Flexion and extension. **34.** A. Supination and adduction. **35.** C. The middle deltoid. **36.** D. Rectus femoris. **37.** B. Lower, middle, and upper. **38.** D. Both B) Sternoclavicular and C) Acromioclavicular. **39.** B. Internal rotation. **40.** D. Abduction.

41. A. Flexion, extension, internal and external rotation, abduction, and adduction. **42.** B. Forward flexion. **43.** B. A large base of support. **44.** C. Sciatic. **45.** A. Ulnar nerve. **46.** D. Atrophy. **47.** A. Outermost. **48.** D. Rhythmic oscillation of the eyeballs. **49.** B. Gastrocnemius and soleus. **50.** C. Spine.

51. F. Answers A) Pubis, B) Ischium, and E) Ilium. **52.** A. Knee flexion and hip extension. **53.** C. Antagonists. **54.** B. Prime movers. **55.** C. Eight. **56.** A. Sensory distribution. **57.** C. The serratus anterior. **58.** A. Forward flexion. **59.** B. A cavity is deeper than a fossa. **60.** B. The middle trapezius.

61. B. Below the tubercles. **62.** A. The pectoralis minor. **63.** C. Palmaris longus versus flexor carpi radialis. **64.** D. Serratur anterior. **65.** B. Posterior deltoid. **66.** C. Abduction–adduction movements take place in a frontal plane.

SECTION II

Theory

Part A

Pediatrics

Select the Most Appropriate Answer

1. The type of cerebral palsy in which there is hearing impairment is one of the following:

    A. Athetoid
    B. Spastic
    C. Ataxic
    D. Flaccid

2. Which of the following normal development theorists is a registered occupational therapist?

    A. Skinner
    B. Maslow
    C. Freud
    D. Grady

3. Spastic cerebral palsy is the result of a lesion in the:

    A. Motor cortex
    B. Spinal cord
    C. Cerebellum
    D. Basal ganglia

4. The pragmatic approach in pediatric occupational therapy (OT) intervention is the same as:

    A. A neurodevelopmental treatment
    B. The orthopedic approach
    C. The rood approach
    D. A mixture of different approaches

5. Which of the following statements is *not* a factor in game leadership?

    A. Involve every child
    B. Give detailed verbal instructions
    C. Consider the safety of the activity
    D. Be aware of activities of the unskilled
    E. Systematic distribution of needed equipment

6. The low organization game formation that requires the least discipline on the part of the leader is:

   A.   Single line
   B.   Shuttle
   C.   Circle
   D.   Relay
   E.   Square

7. A low organization game can be designed:

   A.   To promote motor skills
   B.   To play to win every time
   C.   To elicit cooperative play attitudes
   D.   B and C
   E.   A and C

8. Retarded children require play environments that are:

   A.   Nurturing
   B.   Unstructured
   C.   Structured
   D.   A and C

9. One of the main characteristics of the athetoid cerebral palsied child is:

   A.   Rigidity
   B.   Flaccidity
   C.   Spasticity
   D.   "Snake-like" movements

10. Lordosis is:

   A.   A type of scoliosis
   B.   "Sway back"
   C.   A lateral curvature
   D.   "Hunch back"

11. Within the progression of anatomical maturation, normal growth and development of the human body occur in the following manner:

   A.   Cephalocaudal
   B.   Each child develops at the same pace
   C.   The behavior of a child improves consistently
   D.   Proximal to distal
   E.   A and D

12. The first geometric figure that a child is able to cut with a pair of scissors is the:

    A. Triangle
    B. Square
    C. Circle
    D. Rectangle

13. Within motor accuracy, which of the following elements develops first?

    A. Hand preference
    B. Unilateral
    C. Bilateral
    D. All the above

14. The richest tactile receptors are the:

    A. Feet
    B. Abdomen and neck
    C. Hands and forearms
    D. B and C

15. Within the sequence of normal development, a child recognizes one of the following first:

    A. Linear objects
    B. Two-dimensional objects
    C. Three-dimensional objects
    D. A and C simultaneously

16. If one is right handed, which is/are the dominant hemisphere(s)?

    A. Right
    B. Left
    C. Either A or B
    D. A and B

17. Handedness is normally established:

    A. By 3 years of age
    B. By school age
    C. By preteen years
    D. By 10 years of age

18. The Southern California Motor Accuracy Test was developed by:

    A. Spitz
    B. Piaget
    C. Ayres
    D. Freud

19. The cause of Downs syndrome is:

    A. Chromosomal abnormality
    B. Prematurity
    C. Anoxia
    D. Trauma at birth

20. The following is a behavioral characteristic of a mentally retarded person:

    A. A strong ego
    B. High self-esteem
    C. Self-devaluation
    D. He or she can follow directions easily

21. An apraxic child has a problem with:

    A. Motor accuracy
    B. Kinesthesia
    C. Motor planning
    D. Proprioception

22. A clutterer speaks:

    A. Too slowly
    B. Hesitantly
    C. Too rapidly
    D. A and B

23. Lordosis is an abnormal curvature of the spine characterized by:

    A. A left to right curvature
    B. An exaggerated anterior convexity of the spine
    C. An exaggerated lumbar shifting
    D. A rotation deformity

24. Muscular dystrophy is characterized by:
    A. Progressive degeneration of voluntary musculature
    B. Progressive weakness of voluntary musculature
    C. Voluntary clonus of voluntary musculature
    D. A and C

25. Within Gilfoyle's spatiotemporal adaptation theory, assimilation is:
    A. Sensory reception of stimuli
    B. The body's motor response to stimuli
    C. Discriminating essential elements of a specific behavior
    D. None of the above

26. Aphasia is defined as:
    A. Repetition of what is said
    B. Ability to pursue a single line
    C. Inability of self-expression through speech
    D. Difficult speech due to impairment of the muscles of phonation

27. Position in space is the:
    A. Ability to identify the whole object by seeing only part of it
    B. Ability to know how an object is turned
    C. Ability of the observer to perceive the position of two or more objects in relation to himself or herself and to each other
    D. B and C

28. Echolalia is:
    A. Difficulty in expression of ideas through speech
    B. Defective speech due to impairment of the muscles of phonation
    C. Repetition of what is said but the meaning is not associated with the words
    D. Difficulty in understanding the spoken word

29. Spatial relationships are the:
    A. Ability to follow a moving object with the eyes
    B. Ability to identify the whole object by only seeing part of it
    C. Ability of the observer to perceive the position of two or more objects in relation to himself or herself and to each other
    D. Ability to know how an object is turned

30. Visual tracking is the:
    A. Retention of a visual image
    B. Ability to follow a moving object with the eyes
    C. Impaired ability to estimate distances in muscular acts
    D. Binocular vision

31. When touching a tactile-defensive child, one of the following reactions can be observed:
    A. Intense withdrawal
    B. No response at all
    C. Careful withdrawal
    D. None of the above

32. A child with cerebral palsy has:
    A. A progressive disease
    B. Sensory and/or motor deficits
    C. A contagious disease
    D. A viral infection

33. Equinus feet are:
    A. Turned inward
    B. Flat feet
    C. Only toes touch the floor
    D. Only heels touch the floor

34. Monoplegia is:
    A. Paralysis of one limb
    B. Paralysis of both upper extremities
    C. Paresis of both lower extremities and one upper extremity
    D. Paralysis of both lower extremities

35. Muscular dystrophy results from:
    A. A virus
    B. Trauma at birth
    C. A genetic abnormality
    D. Toxins

36. Play behavior of the normal child during the sensorimotor period characteristically is:

    A. Symbolic
    B. Exploratory
    C. Imitative
    D. Constructive

37. Common behavioral and learning problems seen in children include:

    A. Fear of change
    B. Lack of motivation
    C. Temper tantrums
    D. All the above

38. Statistically it has been proven that the percentage of mental retardation existent in cerebral palsied children is:

    A. Lower than the well population
    B. The same as the normal population
    C. Higher than the well population
    D. 100%

39. A child with spina bifida generally has:

    A. Paraplegia
    B. Quadriplegia
    C. Hemiplegia
    D. Triplegia

40. According to Bobath, weight bearing decreases:

    A. Flaccidity of muscles
    B. Spasticity of muscles
    C. Subluxation of joints
    D. Stiffness of joints

41. During the toilet training stage, the control of the:

    A. Bowel reaches maturity before the bladder
    B. Bladder reaches maturity before the bowel
    C. Bowel and the bladder reach maturity simultaneously

42. Blindism is:
    A. Eye poking
    B. An involuntary oscillation of the eyeballs
    C. A characteristic of the visually impaired
    D. A and C

43. Learning disabilities are neurological dysfunctions that can affect:
    A. Reading and writing
    B. Speech and mathematics
    C. Perceptions, directionality, and motor coordination
    D. All the above

44. According to the Gesell Institute, what is the first geometric form that a child is able to draw?
    A. A triangle
    B. A cross
    C. A circle
    D. A diamond

45. The inability to work mathematical problems is called:
    A. Agnosia
    B. Acalculia
    C. Aphasia
    D. Apraxia

46. Considering normal development, which of the following statements is *not* true?
    A. Reflexive movement precedes voluntary movement
    B. Motor development occurs proximal to distal
    C. Prehension patterns develop in the ulnar–radial direction
    D. Motor development occurs in the caudal–cephalad direction

47. Generally, the patient with cerebral palsy has:
    A. Spastic muscle tone
    B. Flaccid muscle tone
    C. Normal muscle tone
    D. All the above

48. The word dysarthria means:

    A. Inability to speak clearly because of weakness in the muscles of phonation
    B. Inability to recall words and phrases
    C. Inability to understand the spoken word
    D. Inability to recognize objects or symbols

49. The Bobath Approach is one of the following:

    A. Proprioceptive neuromuscular faciliation technique
    B. Neurodevelopmental treatment
    C. Upper and lower extremities synergies
    D. All the above

50. Protective reflexes that are responses to painful stimuli are called:

    A. Crossed extension reflexes
    B. Withdrawal reflexes
    C. Flexion reflexes
    D. B and C

51. A child with a learning disability may be referred to OT because of:

    A. Clumsiness
    B. Muscle weakness
    C. A and B
    D. None of the above

52. In which part of the hand are the sensory receptors more refined?

    A. Fingertip pads
    B. Palm of hand
    C. Dorsum of hand
    D. Dorsum of fingers

53. A procedure called the "Crede Method" is used mainly to teach quadriplegic and paraplegic patients:

    A. Weight shifting
    B. Feeding techniques
    C. Breathing management
    D. Bladder management

54. The positive reaction of the grasp palmar reflex is usually normal for an infant from birth to 3 to 4 months of age. This reaction is produced by the simultaneous occurrence of finger flexion and a strong grasp, which occurs when the therapist applies pressure on the:

    A. Dorsum of the hand
    B. Volar area of the hand on the ulnar side
    C. Fingertips
    D. Volar area of the hand on the radial side

55. The Denver Development Screening Test is used to evaluate:

    A. Speed and accuracy of task performance
    B. Girls only
    C. Developmental delay
    D. IQ only

56. The earlier the OT intervention is performed in a child with a birth dysfunction, the greater the progress potential because:

    A. No injury to the central nervous system has occurred yet
    B. The central nervous system is still immature and primitive patterns are not strongly developed
    C. Not much activity occurs in the central nervous system in a child of such a young age
    D. Psychosocial components have not been damaged

57. During normal development, the learning process occurs in the following pattern:

    A. A child acquires totally new functions at all times
    B. A child acquires higher functions by the modification of lower level responses
    C. Children learn at the same pace
    D. None of the above

58. The detection of motion as related to balance is a sensory awareness skill called:

    A. Ocular control
    B. Auditory
    C. Vestibular
    D. Tactile

59. The unconscious identification of the position of body parts in space is a sensory awareness skill called:

    A. Stereognosis
    B. Kinesthesia
    C. Ocular control
    D. Proprioception

60. The conscious perception of muscular motion, weight, and position is a sensory awareness skill termed:

    A. Kinesthesia
    B. Proprioception
    C. Olfactory
    D. Vestibular

61. Which of the following is/are not characteristic of a learning disabled child?

    A. Hypoactivity and hyperactivity
    B. Incoordination
    C. Overattention and inattention
    D. Physical pain

62. The two main systems used in the theory of sensory integration are:

    A. Vestibular and visual
    B. Tactile and visual
    C. Tactile and vestibular
    D. None of the above

63. Within the hemispheric specialization theory of normal development, it is believed that the two cerebral hemispheres are not functionally similar. Which of the following is *not* a function of the right hemisphere?

    A. Recognition of music
    B. Verbalization
    C. Recognition of art
    D. Recognition of faces

64. Developmental principles and theories have been widely studied by many scientists. A number of occupational therapists have been involved in theoretical approaches to pediatric OT. Which of the following is/was *not* an occupational therapist?

    A. Elnora Gilfoyle
    B. Lela Llorens
    C. Carl Rogers
    D. Jean Ayres

65. Gilfoyle and Grady's spatiotemporal adaptation theory is particularly important in order to understand developmental disabilities. According to this theory, there are four components within the adaptation process. Identify them:

    A. Symbolic activities, developmental activities, sensory activities, and daily life tasks
    B. Exploratory behavior, manipulation behavior, competency behavior, and achievement behavior
    C. Association, accommodation, assimilation, and differentiation
    D. Sensory input, organization, output, and appropriate response

66. Augmentative communication is a technique that can be used with children who have cerebral palsy or other neurological or developmental disorders. Which of the following is *not* a component of augmentative communication?

    A. Echolalia
    B. Gestures
    C. Body language
    D. Audiovisual equipment

67. The word "ataxia" means:

    A. Inability to estimate the necessary range of motion to reach the target
    B. Slurred speech
    C. Lack of order
    D. Decreased resistance to passive movement

68. Visual perceptual skills include:

    A. Form perception and position in space
    B. Visual acuity and graphesthesia
    C. Depth perception and figure/ground perception
    D. A and C

69. When studying the levels of cognitive development according to Piaget, which of the following is considered the lowest development period?

    A. Preoperational
    B. Concrete operational
    C. Sensorimotor
    D. Formal operational

70. Amyotrophic lateral sclerosis is a progressive disease of the:

    A. Peripheral nerve system
    B. Upper motor neuron
    C. Lower motor neuron
    D. B and C

71. Children who are involved in similar activities but are minimally engaged in direct communication are performing:

    A. Solitary play
    B. Cooperative play
    C. Parallel play
    D. Associative play

72. The percentage of emotional dysfunction in children with cerebral palsy is:

    A. Average
    B. Low
    C. Unknown
    D. High

73. Genu varum is the same as:

    A. Club foot
    B. Equinovarus
    C. Bow legs
    D. Equinovalgus

74. In pediatric OT, assessment is a continuing process that allows the therapist to:

    A. Solve problems
    B. Determine goals
    C. Define problems
    D. Interpret data

75. A scooter board is perceived to be a:

    A. Transfer assist unit
    B. Seating apparatus
    C. Mobility mechanism
    D. Positioning device

76. Mentally retarded children have the tendency to display all of the following *except*:
    A. Problems with laterality
    B. Difficulty with spatial relations
    C. Impaired organizational skills of perception stimuli
    D. High intellectual ability

77. Considering the sequence of normal development, which is the first type of movement behavior?
    A. Rolling
    B. Crawling
    C. Creeping
    D. Kneeling

78. A clubfoot can be seen in children with the following conditions *except*:
    A. Poliomyelitis
    B. Spina bifida
    C. Cerebral palsy
    D. Juvenile rheumatoid arthritis

79. The onset of muscular dystrophy is usually:
    A. In old age
    B. In childhood
    C. In adolescence
    D. In young adults

80. All of the following prenatal infections may cause mental retardation *except*:
    A. Syphilis
    B. Influenza
    C. Rubella
    D. Variola

81. Birth injuries may result in the following *except*:
    A. Limitations in learning
    B. Inability to perform activities of daily living independently
    C. Delays in development
    D. Increased interaction with peers

Part B

Physical Dysfunction

Select the Most Appropriate Answer

1. A patient with a cerebrovascular accident (CVA) who neglects the paralyzed extremities displays a type of behavior called:

   A. Regression
   B. Denial
   C. Anxiety
   D. Depression

2. What type of door is more easily handled by a paraplegic individual in a wheelchair?

   A. Sliding door with top and bottom runners
   B. Door that opens toward the individual
   C. Double door that opens from the center toward the individual
   D. Folding door

3. What type of door is more easily opened by a quadriplegic patient?

   A. Sliding door
   B. Pressure mat door
   C. Folding door
   D. Hinged door

4. A therapist may give a handroll to a patient in order to:

   A. Prevent further contractures of the fingers
   B. Prevent finger nails from digging in the palm of the hand
   C. Make cleanliness of the hand easier
   D. All the above

5. The kitchen layout for an individual in a wheelchair should be based on the three-point work triangle. The most efficient layout for the right-handed person arranged from the right to left is:

    A. Sink, cooking facilities, and refrigerator
    B. Refrigerator, sink, and cooking facilities
    C. Cooking facilities, refrigerator, and sink
    D. Sink, refrigerator, and cooking facilities

6. A paraplegic patient in a wheelchair needs:

    A. As much adaptive equipment as possible
    B. More life space than the average person
    C. As much life space as the average person
    D. Many persons helping him or her

7. Receptive aphasia is when:

    A. One cannot express himself or herself
    B. One cannot understand verbal directions
    C. One cannot understand written directions
    D. B and C

8. Communication skills are one of the subdivisions of activities of daily living (ADL) and as such include the:

    A. Ability to read
    B. Ability to use scissors and similar independent items
    C. Ability to listen
    D. Ability to speak
    E. A, C, and D

9. Which of the following is a malignant tumor?

    A. Fibroma
    B. Papilloma
    C. Carcinoma
    D. Lipoma

10. A chondroma is a tumor of the:

    A. Muscles
    B. Cartilage
    C. Skin
    D. Bone

11. A characteristic of a radial nerve injury is the:

    A. Benediction hand
    B. Claw hand
    C. Drop wrist
    D. Waiter's tip position

12. Homonymous hemianopsia is described as:

    A. More disabling than one eye blindness
    B. Most commonly appears with hemiplegia
    C. Refers to the loss of half of the visual field on the same side of each eye
    D. Results in blindness on the same side as the paralysis
    E. All the above
    F. None of the above

13. A static hand splint has:

    A. Moving parts
    B. No moving parts
    C. Both the above
    D. Either A or B

14. An open fracture is also called:

    A. Simple
    B. Greenstick
    C. Comminuted
    D. Compound

15. Traction is an orthopedic treatment procedure that can be defined as a:

    A. Sustained pull
    B. Pull in the proper direction to maintain the alignment of the fragments
    C. Distraction forced on the vertebrae
    D. A and B

16. A closed fracture is referred to as:

    A. Compound
    B. Comminuted
    C. Simple
    D. Transverse

17. One piece of adaptive equipment for a hemiplegic would most likely include a:
    A. Built-up handle
    B. Universal cuff
    C. Rocker knife
    D. Swivel fork

18. A paraplegic is an individual who has paralysis in:
    A. The upper and lower extremities
    B. The area downward from the trunk
    C. One side of the body (left or right)
    D. Lower extremities only

19. A goniometer is an instrument that measures:
    A. Grasping power
    B. The distance between the fingertips and the palmar crease when trying to make a fist
    C. The angles of joints
    D. Edema

20. The initials BTE mean:
    A. Bilateral triphasic equipment
    B. Baltimore treatment equipment
    C. Boston triage equipment
    D. None of the above

21. Generally, a post-hand injury patient should:
    A. Hold the hand motionless
    B. Exercise the free joints as much as possible
    C. Exercise adjacent joints to the cast
    D. B and C

22. Fluidotherapy is a:
    A. Whirlpool treatment
    B. Physical medicine modality
    C. Hand carpometacarpal unit
    D. Coban wrap technique

23. Hemiplegia is the total paralysis of:

    A. Both legs
    B. Both arms
    C. One side of the body (right or left)
    D. Only one arm
    E. Only one leg
    F. Both arms and legs

24. The main objective of passive exercise of the shoulder is:

    A. To increase the stiffness of the shoulder
    B. To keep the shoulder free of contractures
    C. To increase spasticity of the shoulder
    D. To decrease flaccidity of the shoulder

25. A patient with a greenstick fracture has:

    A. A splintered fracture
    B. An oblique fracture
    C. A transverse fracture
    D. A bone that fractures incompletely

26. Following a fracture, there are several stages of bone repair. The first healing stage is:

    A. Remodeling
    B. Callus formation
    C. Hematoma
    D. Recanalization

27. Bouchard's nodes are usually observed in which of the following joints:

    A. Radioulnar
    B. Proximal interphalangeals
    C. Intercarpals
    D. Distal interphalangeals

28. Which of the following is *not* considered a work-simplification technique?

    A. Hiring someone to do the task
    B. Duplicating cleaning agents for use in the bathroom and in the kitchen
    C. Standing rather than sitting when ironing
    D. Air drying dishes rather than drying them with a towel

29. A patient with a median nerve injury that occurred 3 inches above the distal wrist crease will have difficulty with:

    A. Supination and pronation
    B. Finger extension
    C. Wrist extension
    D. Thumb opposition

30. The rheumatic disease that starts in the sacroiliac joints and spreads upward leading to the fusion of the spine is called:

    A. Osteoarthritis
    B. Rheumatoid arthritis
    C. Scleroderma
    D. Ankylosing spondylitis

31. If an individual has a burn involving the superficial layers of the skin, the certified occupational therapy assistant (COTA) can say that he or she has:

    A. A first-degree burn
    B. A third-degree burn
    C. An erythema
    D. A second-degree burn

32. One of the following is *not* a dysfunction of the central nervous system:

    A. Rheumatoid arthritis
    B. A spinal cord injury
    C. Parkinson's disease
    D. Multiple sclerosis

33. The most common etiologic factor of a CVA is:

    A. Ischemia
    B. An embolism
    C. A vasospasm
    D. Thrombosis

34. The rheumatic disease that is characterized by overproduction of uric acid is:

    A. Scleroderma
    B. Gouty arthritis
    C. Ankylosing spondylitis
    D. Osteoarthritis

35. Which of the following is contraindicated in the treatment of the arthritic patient?

    A. Energy conservation
    B. Joint protection
    C. Maintenance of range of motion (ROM) as much as possible
    D. Passive ROM during the acute stage

36. Rheumatoid arthritis usually occurs in:

    A. Young adulthood
    B. Late adulthood
    C. Infancy
    D. Adolescence

37. Osteoarthritis usually occurs in this population:

    A. Young adults
    B. Late adulthood
    C. Infants
    D. Adolescents

38. According to the neurodevelopmental treatment developed by Bobath and Bobath, which of the following is indicated for the hemiplegic patient?

    A. Weight bearing on the involved side
    B. Approach the patient from the involved side
    C. Elongation of the involved side
    D. All the above

39. The word flaccidity means:

    A. Hypertonicity of the muscles
    B. Hypotonicity of the muscles
    C. Rigidity of the muscles
    D. Unwanted resistance

40. Which of the following is a main concern in the rehabilitation of a spinal cord injured patient?

    A. Prevention of decubitus
    B. Heavy resistive exercises
    C. Promote dependency
    D. Low fluid intake

41. Function(s) of splinting include:
    A. To prevent contractures
    B. To increase function
    C. To increase joint ROM
    D. Joint protection
    E. All the above

42. A quadriplegic patient who has his or her wrist extension graded good (4) may benefit from which of the following splints?
    A. Tenodesis hand splint
    B. Resting pan hand splint
    C. Cock-up hand splint
    D. Opponens hand splint

43. The word "spasticity" means:
    A. Hypotonicity of muscles
    B. Hypertonicity of muscles
    C. "Floppy" muscles
    D. Rigid muscles

44. When planning the treatment of an injured hand, the therapist must know that the key joint(s) in the mechanics of the hand is/are:
    A. Proximal interphalangeal joints (PIPJs)
    B. Distal interphalangeal joints (DIPJs)
    C. Wrist joint
    D. Intercarpal joints

45. If a patient has third-degree burns, it means:
    A. Only blistering is present
    B. There is slight redness of the skin
    C. There is destruction of the entire thickness of the skin
    D. There is a large area of damage

46. When a COTA reads in the patient's chart that the right tricep is graded zero, he or she will expect that elbow extension is:
    A. Flaccid
    B. Spastic
    C. Rigid
    D. Hypercontractile

47. The multiple sclerotic patient may have a speech impediment called:
    A. Stutter
    B. Aphasia
    C. Clutter
    D. Scanned speech

48. A movement totally performed by the patient through the full range is called:
    A. Passive motion
    B. Active motion
    C. Assistive motion
    D. Passive-assistive motion

49. Usually the position of the spastic hemiplegic patient's upper extremity is described as follows:
    A. Shoulder externally rotated and adducted; elbow, wrist, and fingers flexed
    B. Shoulder internally rotated and adducted; elbow, wrist, and fingers flexed
    C. Shoulder internally rotated and abducted; elbow, wrist, and fingers flexed
    D. Shoulder externally rotated and abducted; elbow, wrist, and fingers extended

50. The main deformity that may occur in the involved upper extremity of the hemiplegic patient who does not receive treatment is:
    A. "Claw hand"
    B. Flexion contracture of wrist
    C. "Frozen shoulder"
    D. Contracture of the elbow

51. In the rehabilitation process of the hemiplegic patient, the most difficult shoulder movement to be regained is:
    A. External rotation
    B. Internal rotation
    C. Flexion
    D. Extension

52. The specific phonation treatment for aphasic patients is best accomplished by:
    A. An occupational therapist
    B. A physical therapist
    C. A speech pathologist
    D. An audiologist

53. A painful shoulder with edema in the hand is considered this type of condition:

    A. Neuritis
    B. Osteoporosis
    C. Shoulder-hand syndrome
    D. Rheumatoid arthritis

54. The loss of blood supply to a body part is called:

    A. Infarction
    B. Anemia
    C. Thrombus
    D. Ischemia

55. During the phase of "phantom limb," the individual with an amputation:

    A. Actively feels the amputated body part
    B. Is aware of heat and cold
    C. Is aware of pain
    D. All the above

56. The voluntary opening of the terminal device of an above elbow prosthesis can be elicited through:

    A. Shoulder flexion
    B. Shoulder extension
    C. Scapula protraction
    D. Scapula adduction

57. Poliomyelitis is a dysfunction of the:

    A. Dorsal root ganglia
    B. Posterior horn cells
    C. Peripheral nerves
    D. Anterior horn cells

58. The detachable desk arms of a wheelchair are of the utmost importance for:

    A. Facilitation of wheelchair mobility
    B. Sitting with good positioning patterns close to a table
    C. Supporting arms while propelling the wheelchair
    D. Sliding board transfers

59. Ambulation of a wheelchair client requires specific architectural modifications for doorways. According to Trombly, the correct door width measurement should be at least:
    A. 32 in.
    B. 34 in.
    C. 31 in.
    D. 36 in.

60. Generally, a static hand splint should hold the wrist in the:
    A. Functional position
    B. Flexion position
    C. Anatomical position
    D. Position of rest

61. Considering associated reactions, which of the following facilitates a flexion reaction in the involved hemiplegic upper extremity?
    A. Resist flexion in uninvolved upper extremity
    B. Resist flexion in involved upper extremity
    C. Resist abduction in uninvolved upper extremity
    D. Resist adduction in involved upper extremity

62. Within the proprioceptive neuromuscular facilitation approach, a loud command will elicit a:
    A. Quick motor response
    B. Moderate motor response
    C. Minimal motor response
    D. Symmetrical motor response

63. From which of the following statements can the therapist assume that an individual has a perceptual impairment?
    A. A hearing impaired person who is unable to attach a meaning to a sound
    B. A visually impaired person who has poor visual acuity
    C. A person with good visual acuity who cannot match shapes or objects
    D. A person who cannot distinguish the different tastes of food

64. When the ROM of an active antigravity movement is less than the ROM of a passive movement, the therapist can conclude that there is most likely a problem with:
    A. Muscle strength
    B. Muscle sensitivity
    C. Muscle coordination
    D. Muscle endurance

65. What is the function of the lumbrical bar attachment on a hand splint?
    A. It prevents hyperextension of the metacarpophalangeal joints (MCPJs)
    B. It decreases flexion of the MCPJs
    C. It increases flexion of the MCPJs
    D. It increases extension of the MCPJs

66. The function of the mobile arm support is to help weak:
    A. Trunk and shoulder muscles
    B. Shoulder and elbow muscles
    C. Hand and wrist muscles
    D. Shoulder muscles

67. The primary objective of the resting pan hand splint is to:
    A. Limit active movement
    B. Limit strength
    C. Conserve energy
    D. Keep good positioning

68. A patient accomplishes active shoulder flexion while standing, but is unable to complete the full ROM without help. This type of exercise is termed:
    A. Isotonic assistive
    B. Passive assistive
    C. Isometric
    D. Isotonic

69. The following components are considered in the assessment of occupational performance tasks:
    A. Perceptual skills
    B. Motor skills
    C. Cognitive skills
    D. Judgment about capabilities
    E. All the above
    F. A, B, and C

70. When a patient who suffered a head injury is aroused only through vigorous stimulation, the level of consciousness is referred to as:
    A. Stupor
    B. Clouding of consciousness
    C. Coma
    D. Obtundity

71. Which of the following is not an example of a perceptual function?

    A. Attention span
    B. Ability to cross the midline
    C. Neglect of one extremity
    D. Space relationship

72. The flexion of the PIPJ and extension of the DIPJ is a deformity termed:

    A. Swan neck
    B. Ulnar drift
    C. Boutonniere
    D. Mallet finger

73. Which type of population seems more at risk for hip fractures?

    A. Elderly men
    B. Female children
    C. Elderly women
    D. Young adult men

74. The most common etiologic factor of low back pain is:

    A. Vertebrae malalignment
    B. Ruptured disk
    C. Facet disrelationships
    D. Soft tissue strain

75. What are the main symptoms of a Parkinson's disease patient?

    A. Euphoria and impaired long-term memory
    B. Tremors, rigidity, and slowness of movement
    C. Depression and impaired long-term memory
    D. Depression and impaired short-term memory

76. The slowing down of a spontaneous motor response is defined as:

    A. Bradykinesia
    B. Kinesthesia
    C. Rigidity
    D. Akinesia

77. What materials, considered low temperature, can be heated in hot water and molded directly onto the patient's skin?

    A. Orthoplast, polyform, and aquaplast
    B. Kidex, plastazote, and aquaplast
    C. Royalite, orthoplast, and kidex
    D. Aquaplast, orthoplast, and kidex

78. The highest incidence of head injury most likely occurs in the following age group:

    A. 21 to 36 years old
    B. 26 to 40 years old
    C. 15 to 29 years old
    D. 11 to 25 years old

79. According to the Rancho Los Amigos Scale of Head Injury, a patient who responds inconsistently and belatedly to stimuli is at level:

    A. IV
    B. VI
    C. III
    D. II

80. The distribution of rheumatoid arthritis is more likely to follow a specific pattern that is:

    A. Unilateral in the upper extremities
    B. Bilateral asymmetrical
    C. Bilateral symmetrical
    D. Sometimes B other times C

81. A patient who is completely flaccid needs this type of exercise:

    A. Active
    B. Passive
    C. Passive assistive
    D. Active assistive

82. According to occupational therapy (OT) experts, the major component regarding the patient's returning to work after an injury is the:

    A. Level of recovery achieved
    B. Patient's educational background
    C. Severity of the injury
    D. Degree of the patient's motivation

83. When a therapist is constructing a hand splint that gives support to the wrist, he or she must extend it to the length of the forearm for appropriate leverage, approximately:

    A. One half of the forearm
    B. Two thirds of the forearm
    C. Three fourths of the forearm
    D. The total length of the forearm

84. What type of leg rests are appropriate for reclining wheelchairs?

    A. Elevating
    B. Swing around detachable
    C. Fixed
    D. Detachable

85. When performing accurate assessments, the evaluation tools should be valid, reliable, and:

    A. Easy to score
    B. Easy to administer
    C. Easy to understand by the patient
    D. Sensitive enough to detect minor changes

86. A patient is diagnosed with a spinal cord injury at the C5 level. What group of muscles has functional potential?

    A. The supinator, the biceps, and the three portions of the deltoid
    B. The pectoralis major, the triceps, and the three portions of the deltoid
    C. The biceps, the three portions of the trapezius, and serratus anterior
    D. The serratus anterior, the latissimus dorsi, and the three portions of the trapezius

87. "Pill-rolling" tremors are an example of:

    A. Action tremors
    B. Resting tremors
    C. Intention tremors
    D. Physiological tremors

88. Which of the following is a symptom of an ulnar nerve injury?

    A. The inability to abduct the wrist
    B. The inability to adduct the wrist
    C. The inability to extend the wrist
    D. The inability to oppose the thumb

89. During the aging process, the intervertebral disc loses:

    A. Water
    B. Elastic properties
    C. Permeability
    D. All the above

90. Most patients with spinal cord dysfunctions that result in quadriplegia receive lesions at which of the following levels?

    A. C2 to C3
    B. C4 to C5
    C. C3 to C4
    D. C5 to C6

91. An individual has an above elbow prosthesis. Of all the prosthetic components, which is the most significant?

    A. A triceps pad
    B. A wrist unit
    C. A terminal device
    D. A cable system

92. Which of the following is characteristic of a patient with multiple sclerosis:

    A. Bradykinesia
    B. Resting tremors
    C. Rigidity
    D. Remissions and exacerbations

93. Individuals who, as a rule, arrive late to work, cannot meet deadlines, and do not follow instructions should attend:

    A. Work activities programs
    B. Vocational training programs
    C. Prevocational programs
    D. Work adjustment programs

94. Hyperextension of the PIPJ and flexion of the DIPJ is a deformity called:

    A. Ulnar drift
    B. Boutonniere
    C. Mallet finger
    D. Swan neck

95. Unilateral neglect generally occurs in:

    A. Right hemiparesia

    B. Tactile dysfunction

    C. Left hemiparesia

    D. A and C

96. The following may be a sign of a heart attack:

    A. Nystagmus

    B. Shortness of breath

    C. Numbness of the arm

    D. Chest pain or pressure

    E. B and D

97. The most functional prehension pattern occurs when the wrist is in:

    A. Flexion

    B. Pronation

    C. Adduction

    D. Dorsiflexion

98. The typical position of a hemiplegic patient's lower extremity is:

    A. Hip flexion and internal rotation, knee flexion, ankle plantar flexion and inversion, and toes flexion

    B. Hip internal rotation, abduction and extension, knee extension, ankle plantar flexion and inversion, and toes flexion

    C. Hip external rotation and adduction, knee flexion, and ankle and toes flexion

    D. Hip flexion and internal rotation, knee extension, and ankle dorsiflexion and eversion

99. Kitchen counters in ADL areas in OT clinics have to be accessible to wheelchair clients; therefore, they must be positioned at one of the following heights:

    A. 26½ in.

    B. 29½ in.

    C. 32 in.

    D. 34 in.

100. The instrument used to measure grasping power is called a:

    A. Sphygmometer

    B. Dynamometer

    C. Goniometer

    D. Pinch gauge

101. Identify the instrument shown in the picture (Figure 2-1):

    A. Pinch gauge
    B. Spirometer
    C. Dynamometer
    D. Goniometer

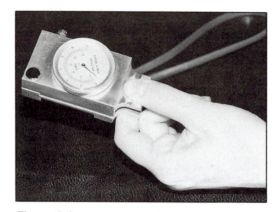

Figure 2-1.

102. Identify the instrument shown in the picture (Figure 2-2):

    A. Pinch gauge
    B. Spirometer
    C. Goniometer
    D. Dynamometer

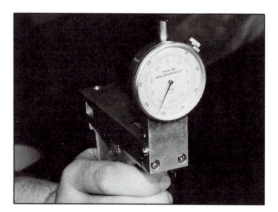

Figure 2-2.

103. Identify the instrument shown in the picture (Figure 2-3):

    A. Pinch gauge
    B. Dynamometer
    C. Goniometer
    D. Aesthesiometer

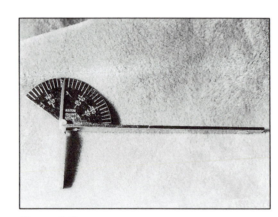

Figure 2-3.

104. The hand splint in the picture is which one of the following (Figure 2-4)?

    A. Resting pan hand splint
    B. Cock-up hand splint
    C. Opponens splint
    D. Tenodesis hand splint

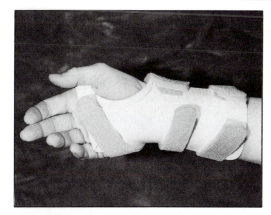

Figure 2-4.

105. Identify the hand splint shown in the picture (Figure 2-5):

    A. Resting pan hand splint
    B. Cock-up hand splint
    C. Opponens splint
    D. Tenodesis hand splint

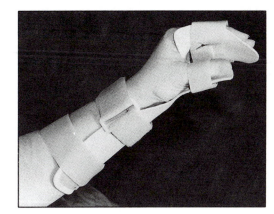

Figure 2-5.

106. Identify the hand splint shown in the picture (Figure 2-6):

    A. Resting pan hand splint
    B. Cock-up hand splint
    C. Opponens splint
    D. Tenodesis hand splint

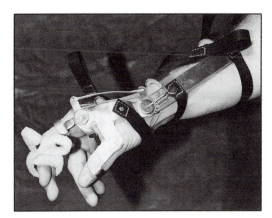

Figure 2-6.

107. Identify the hand splint shown in the picture (Figure 2-7):

   A. Resting pan hand splint
   B. Cock-up hand splint
   C. Opponens splint
   D. Tenodesis hand splint

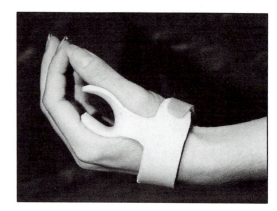

Figure 2-7.

108. The following are characteristics of rheumatoid arthritis in its later stages, *except*:

   A. Contractures of soft tissues
   B. Ulnar deviation of fingers
   C. Heberden's nodes
   D. Muscular atrophy

109. The following are characteristics of osteoarthritis, *except*:

   A. Sudden onset
   B. Rest relieves pain
   C. Bony spurs
   D. Bouchard's nodes

110. Dysphagia is:

   A. Inflammation of the mouth
   B. The loss of a desire to eat
   C. Incoordinated movements
   D. Difficulty in swallowing

111. An osteotomy is:

   A. Surgical immobilization of a joint
   B. Bone infection
   C. Debridement
   D. Surgical sectioning of a bone

112. Arthroplasty is defined as:

    A. An operation associated with osteomyelitis
    B. A condition characterized by bony spurring
    C. An operation to restore mobility to a stiffened joint
    D. A surgical procedure to fuse a joint

113. Which of these bone tumors is malignant?

    A. Osteoma
    B. Osteochondroma
    C. Chondroma
    D. Osteosarcoma

114. Atrophy of the muscles of the thenar eminence indicates most likely an injury of the:

    A. Median nerve
    B. Musculocutaneous nerve
    C. Ulnar nerve
    D. Radial nerve

115. When an organ is removed, which suffix would be attached to the surgical procedure?

    A. Ostomy
    B. Ography
    C. Ectomy
    D. Oscopy

116. A surgery commonly used to remove benign tumors in the uterus is a:

    A. Myectomy
    B. Cystectomy
    C. Nephrectomy
    D. Hysterectomy

117. The following are consequences of a heart attack, *except*:

    A. Activity level declines
    B. Muscle strength decreases
    C. Endurance increases
    D. Lifestyle abruptly changes

118. One of these dysfunctions is *not* called a neuromuscular disease:
    A.   Amyotrophic lateral sclerosis
    B.   Scleroderma
    C.   Multiple sclerosis
    D.   Myasthenia gravis

119. Which of these statements is *not* true when considering the etiology of rheumatoid arthritis?
    A.   It initially affects the small peripheral joints
    B.   The average age of onset is approximately 40 years old
    C.   It is characterized by joint wear and tear
    D.   It affects women more than men

Part C

Psychosocial Dysfunction

Select the Most Appropriate Answer

1. When dealing with death, the adolescent may go through the following sequence of stages:
    A. Anger—denial—bargaining—depression—acceptance
    B. Denial—anger—depression—bargaining—acceptance
    C. Depression—denial—anger—bargaining—acceptance
    D. Denial—anger—bargaining—depression—acceptance

2. The word anorexia means:
    A. Nausea and vomiting
    B. Overeating
    C. Loss of appetite
    D. Fear of eating

3. A neurotic individual may use anxiety in the form of physical impairment to avoid unacceptable behavior. This type of reaction is termed:
    A. Exaggerated dependency
    B. Reaction formation
    C. Conversion reaction
    D. Aggression and hostility

4. Which of the following is *not* considered a characteristic of a manic patient?
    A. Docile
    B. Egocentric
    C. Distractable
    D. Expansive

5. When a therapist needs to establish an interpersonal relationship with a manic patient, the professional should encourage:
    A. Praise
    B. Decision making
    C. Verbal recognition of the patient's feelings
    D. Meeting dependency needs

6. Which of the following is inappropriate for a depressed patient?
   A. Short-term activities
   B. Structured activities
   C. Unstructured activities
   D. Simplified activities

7. The convulsions of a grand mal seizure that occur in the epileptic patient have:
   A. A clonic phase
   B. A tonic phase
   C. A stable phase
   D. A and B

8. Nonverbal communication in many circumstances could indicate that the patient:
   A. Is explaining something he cannot put into words
   B. Is depressed
   C. Does not want to communicate verbally
   D. All of the above

9. In general, communication includes:
   A. A verbal area
   B. A nonverbal area
   C. The written word
   D. Body language
   E. All the above

10. A false belief that cannot be altered by reasoning is called:
    A. Disillusion
    B. Delusion
    C. Illusion
    D. Self-abasement

11. Sensory perceptions that are *not* based on objective stimulation are called:
    A. Insight
    B. Disillusions
    C. Hallucinations
    D. Imagination

12. A patient who constantly keeps a specific position is diagnosed as:

    A. Catatonic
    B. Negativistic
    C. Depressed
    D. Resistive

13. Bisexuality is a concept that evolves from which stage of development:

    A. Oedipal
    B. Anal
    C. Oral
    D. Adolescence

14. Psychodrama is a treatment technique used in mental illness for the purpose of:

    A. Release therapy
    B. Remotivation
    C. Reality orientation
    D. Reorientation orientation

15. Within normal development, the oral stage is considered:

    A. A period of avoidance
    B. A period of tolerance
    C. A time of dependency
    D. A time of morality

16. This type of dysfunction may occur following the death of a loved one:

    A. Reactive depression
    B. Postpartum depression
    C. Involuntional melancholia
    D. Bipolar disorder

17. The inability to deal with reality is termed:

    A. Anxiety reaction
    B. Phobic reaction
    C. Psychosis
    D. Neurotic reaction

18. Auditory hallucinations are disturbances in:
    A. Object relationships
    B. Perception
    C. The affective domain
    D. Memory

19. The term used to describe distortions of the body image and feelings of unreality is:
    A. Transference
    B. Derealization
    C. Suppression
    D. Depersonalization

20. The term superego can be defined as:
    A. The result of learning that what feels good really is bad
    B. Ethics, self-criticism
    C. Group status for overwhelming individual weaknesses
    D. Polarized attitudes

21. Underactivity is a disturbance common in:
    A. Depression
    B. Affective reactions
    C. Mania
    D. Catatonia

22. Overactivity is a disturbance common in:
    A. Affective reactions
    B. Schizophrenia
    C. Mania
    D. Paranoia

23. A sound produced by an object was incorrectly interpreted as being produced by a human voice. This perception disorder is called:
    A. "Deja Vu"
    B. Illusion
    C. Disillusion
    D. Negativism

24. Depression is an impairment of one of the following:

    A. Instinct
    B. Affective domain
    C. Consciousness
    D. Thought

25. The phenomenon of automatic repetition of words or phrases that were spoken by someone else is termed:

    A. Echolalia
    B. Projection
    C. Echomania
    D. Echopraxia

26. Antisocial behavior is characteristic of:

    A. Affective disorders
    B. Organic mental disorders
    C. Eating disorders
    D. Conduct disorders

27. Sensory integration is the:

    A. Capacity to manage oneself in conducting daily affairs
    B. Individual's recognition of self
    C. Processing of sensory information so an individual can act in the environment
    D. Ability to work and play in the presence of others

28. Reality testing means one of the following:

    A. The environment is considered objectively
    B. Acceptable rules or standards for normal behavior
    C. Reasonable understanding of self and others
    D. Pervasive sustained emotion

29. Which of the following is *not* a type of dyadic interaction:

    A. Friendships
    B. A task group
    C. Intimate relationships
    D. Superior–subordinate relationship

30. Cohesiveness is a crucial component in a group. How can this be facilitated?

    A. Reality testing
    B. Antigroup roles
    C. Intermember dissimilarities
    D. Intermember similarities

31. Dyadic interaction means:

    A. When one engages in interaction with another
    B. The ability to locate oneself in one's environment
    C. The retention and storage of information for further use
    D. When one engages in interaction with a group of people

32. Jane has come to occupational therapy with several problems related to activities of daily living and self-worth. She must apply for welfare to sustain herself. According to Maslow's hierarchy of needs, which need must be satisfied first?

    A. Belonging—love
    B. Self-actualization
    C. Physiological
    D. Self-esteem

33. A certified occupational therapy assistant is working in a goal setting group. Each patient must have very specific goals that have to be:

    A. Measurable
    B. Achievable
    C. Understandable
    D. All the above

34. "You are hostile to me because I may remind you of your mother." This statement is:

    A. Condescending
    B. Punishing
    C. Interpreting
    D. "Passing the buck"

35. "Sorry, I didn't hear you, my mind wandered" may be interpreted as:

    A. "You're not as healthy as I am"
    B. "You're not as sensitive as I am"
    C. "I'll get you for ignoring me"
    D. "Your feelings are unimportant"

36. Communication is a two-way affair. Besides expressing our feelings to others, we must permit others to express their feelings to us. Which of the following is an inappropriate approach?

    A. Empathic response leads
    B. "Passing the buck"
    C. Condescending attitude
    D. Incredulity

37. The etiologic factor of neuroses is one of the following:

    A. Depression
    B. Conflict
    C. Anxiety
    D. Disorientation

38. Making a client familiar with his or her surroundings within the acute psychiatric clinic will satisfy what type of needs?

    A. Self-actualization
    B. Cognitive
    C. Safety
    D. Aesthetic

39. Mental health includes:

    A. Social well-being
    B. Adaptation
    C. Personal satisfaction
    D. Sense of well-being
    E. All the above

40. Free association is defined as:

    A. The analyst's attitude toward the patient
    B. The emotional reaction of the patient toward the analyst
    C. One's inner tensions are expressed symbolically and disguised
    D. An unconscious effort to evade

41. Self-esteem is:

    A. A negative self-concept
    B. Thinking well of oneself
    C. Feelings of inadequacy
    D. An awareness of shortcomings

42. Delusions are examples of an impairment of:

    A. Judgment
    B. Perception
    C. Memory
    D. Thought

43. People greatly influence the "shaping" process of one's self-concept. This process occurs in two different ways:

    A. Social comparison
    B. Linear communication
    C. Empathic leads
    D. Reflected appraisal
    E. A and D
    F. B and C

44. In considering a patient, which of the following areas should a therapist use in the holistic health concept?

    A. Biological, natural, sociocultural
    B. Psychological, spiritual, organic
    C. Spiritual, intellectual, organic
    D. Sociocultural, biological, aging

45. Mental illness is:

    A. Response to stress
    B. Interference with ability to cope
    C. Ambivalence
    D. Maladaptive behavior

46. Denial is a coping mechanism that can be detected in which of the following statements?

    A. A man with intense hostile feelings becomes a lumberjack
    B. Instead of discussing a problem, the person pretends it doesn't exist
    C. A husband is angry at his supervisor; he comes home and yells at his wife
    D. One avoids facing an unpleasant truth by reacting in exactly the opposite manner

47. Amnesia is an impairment of which of the following:

    A. Judgment
    B. Perception
    C. Memory
    D. Affective domain

48. Ego is a personality structure with one of the following characteristics:

    A. Demands immediate gratification of desires
    B. Acts as the repressing part of the personality
    C. Operates on the "reality principle"
    D. The "observing portion" of the personality

49. Assessment of the interpersonal component of performance determines the individual's

    A. Ability to cope with stress
    B. Ability to relate to others
    C. Inability to separate reality from fantasy
    D. Inability to accept criticism

50. When assessing one's leisure time use, the therapist needs to determine:

    A. The person's amount of work time versus leisure time
    B. The person's enjoyment interests
    C. The person's work habits
    D. The number of friends an individual has

51. The existence of opposing feelings and attitudes toward the same object is termed:

    A. Depression
    B. Perception
    C. Disorientation
    D. Ambivalence

52. The need to assess addicted clients for sensory integrative dysfunctions is based on:

    A. Low self-esteem
    B. An inability to cope with stressful situations
    C. A deficient ability to process information internally
    D. Poor working habits

53. When working in a hospice program, the therapist should realize that Americans generally cope with death by:

    A. Using avoidance, denial, and repudiation
    B. Making plans to be carried out after their death
    C. Asking relatives to help them make plans
    D. Spending a great deal of time with a member of the clergy to help them accept death

54. Behaviors that oppose what the patient really wants are called:
    A. Compensation
    B. Rationalization
    C. Reaction formation
    D. Dissociation

55. An epileptic seizure of the grand mal type has one of the following characteristics:
    A. Complete and sudden loss of consciousness
    B. Presence of a clonic phase and absence of a tonic phase
    C. Presence of a tonic phase and absence of a clonic phase
    D. Alteration of awareness connected with cognitive skills

56. Hypnosis is a type of psychotherapy defined in one sense as:
    A. A treatment method for unmanageable anxiety
    B. An unconscious effort to evade
    C. An emotional reliving of stressful situations
    D. A behavior control technique

57. The etiologic factor of Korsakoff's psychosis is one of the following:
    A. Metabolic imbalances
    B. Genetic factor
    C. Vitamin C deficiency
    D. Thiamine deficiency

58. Coping mechanisms are emotions and behaviors that enable individuals to adjust to problems. One of the following is *not* a coping mechanism:
    A. Displacement
    B. Delusion
    C. Projection
    D. Rationalization

59. One who systematically opposes and resists any type of suggestion is displaying:
    A. Negativism
    B. Denial
    C. Compensation
    D. Dissociation

60. Attention is the process by which an individual voluntarily focuses and distracts from specific mental activities. This process is:

    A. Identification
    B. Unconscious
    C. Subconscious
    D. Selective

61. A person has poor adaption skills, is unable to accept responsibility, and shies away from any demands set upon him or her. Which of the following personality patterns fits this description?

    A. Paranoid
    B. Bipolar
    C. Inadequate
    D. Schizoid

62. Short attention span is a disorder of:

    A. Perception
    B. Judgment
    C. Intellectual function
    D. Memory

63. When an individual is overwhelmed by a crisis, he or she may develop one of the following in order to resolve the situation:

    A. Compensation
    B. Sublimation
    C. Conversion reaction
    D. Regression

64. Phobic thoughts are:

    A. Irrational fears
    B. Rational fears
    C. Obsessions
    D. Ruminations

65. A thought disorder with a nonmeaningful persistent repetition of a specific idea is termed:

    A. Affectivity
    B. Perseveration
    C. Lability
    D. Flight of ideas

66. One of the following is characteristic of a client with psychosis:

    A. Generally regards himself or herself as ill

    B. Has difficulty maintaining socially acceptable behavior

    C. Is painfully aware of his or her own failure to live up to society's expectations

    D. Makes an effort to maintain socially acceptable behavior

67. Psychoanalysis is a treatment technique used with the mentally ill that was originated by:

    A. Meyer

    B. Ayres

    C. Freud

    D. Adler

68. Which of the following is characteristic of the phallic stage?

    A. Period of complete dependence

    B. Search for personal identity

    C. Concern arises regarding physical differences between boys and girls

    D. Occupational choices are generally made

69. Delirium tremens is a dysfunction that results from:

    A. An endocrine imbalance

    B. Taking an occasional alcoholic drink

    C. Drinking over a long period of time

    D. Sudden withdrawal of alcohol from a chronic alcoholic

70. Confabulation is a disturbance of which of the following:

    A. Perception

    B. Memory

    C. Judgment

    D. Thought content

71. In psychoanalytic therapy, the term countertransference means:

    A. The tentative explanation of the patient's feelings and behaviors

    B. The therapist's attitudes toward the patient

    C. The unconscious effort to evade

    D. The patient's emotional reactions toward therapist

72. The drug Valium is categorized under one of the following:

    A. Antidepressant
    B. Anticholinergic
    C. Antianxiety
    D. Antipsychotic

73. The type of psychotherapy which aims to structure the environment so the child can learn adaptive acceptable behavior patterns is termed:

    A. Play therapy
    B. Art therapy
    C. Reality therapy
    D. Behavior therapy

74. The diagnostic and statistic manual of mental disorders (DSM-III-R) is a source used to recognize and describe emotional and behavioral disorders of infancy, childhood, and adolescence. This manual was published by the:

    A. American Medical Association
    B. American Occupational Therapy Association
    C. American Psychiatric Association
    D. None of the above

75. Thorazine is one of the somatic therapy drugs commonly used in psychiatry. This drug is an:

    A. Antipsychotic agent
    B. Antimanic agent
    C. Antidepressant agent
    D. Antianxiety agent

76. Euphoria is a dysfunction of which of the following:

    A. Judgment
    B. Consciousness
    C. Thought content
    D. Affect

77. The word narcissism means:

    A. Feeling safe from impulses
    B. Intense love and dependency upon parents
    C. Self-admiration

78. Chemical dependency may cause all of the following, *except:*

    A. Increased stress among family and friends
    B. Increased social interests
    C. Decreased self-esteem
    D. Decreased leisure activities

79. Which one of the following does the American Occupational Therapy Association consider a consequence of mental illness?

    A. Inadequate job skills
    B. Stress-free everyday living
    C. Appropriate social interactions
    D. Ease in expressing emotions

80. A client with a passive–aggressive personality will exhibit all of the following, *except:*

    A. Procrastination
    B. Pouting
    C. Indecisiveness
    D. Stubborness

81. Oversuspicion and delusion of persecution are characteristics of a patient with:

    A. Passive–dependent behavior
    B. Catatonia
    C. Hebephrenia
    D. Paranoia

82. The term that describes abnormal fear of heights is:

    A. Acrophobia
    B. Agorophobia
    C. Hydrophobia
    D. Claustrophobia

83. A client who displays psychotic–paranoid reactions uses which of the following defense mechanism excessively?

    A. Projection
    B. Rationalization
    C. Reaction formation
    D. Sublimation

84. Compulsive personalities include:

    A. Bipolar behavior
    B. Perfectionism
    C. Suspiciousness
    D. Antisocial behavior

85. An individual with a neurosis who acts as if obvious reality does not exist is using the defense mechanism of:

    A. Projection
    B. Introjection
    C. Regression
    D. Denial

86. A client who tends to show inner psychological conflicts through somatic disturbances most likely displays:

    A. Conversion reaction
    B. Denial
    C. Anxiety reaction
    D. Dissociative reaction

87. Ego is the part of the personality that:

    A. Develops feelings of guilt
    B. Exists at birth
    C. Makes voluntary decisions
    D. Differentiates between right and wrong

88. The portion of the personality termed id contains one of the following:

    A. A guilt complex
    B. Basic instinctual drives
    C. A censorship mechanism
    D. Control of voluntary movement

89. The developmental stage in which the personality has its first experience with authority is:

    A. Anal
    B. Adolescence
    C. Latent
    D. Oedipal

90. Which of these is *not* a defense mechanism?

    A. Depression

    B. Projection

    C. Sublimation

    D. Regression

91. All of these characteristics are typical of a passive–dependent individual, *except:*

    A. Emotional dependency

    B. Obstructionism

    C. Overtly displaying aggression

    D. Poor self-confidence

92. A condition in which a person has abnormal fear of closed spaces is called:

    A. Agorophobia

    B. Claustrophobia

    C. Acrophobia

    D. Photophobia

93. A client who suddenly refers a paralysis of the right lower extremity without an organic cause is most likely expressing:

    A. A denial reaction

    B. A dissociative reaction

    C. A conversion reaction

    D. An anxiety reaction

94. Which of these statements does *not* apply to psychosis?

    A. The presence of severe disorganization of the personality

    B. May be precipitated by toxic factors

    C. The patient retains reality-testing functions

    D. The client loses his or her reality-testing functions

95. One of these defense mechanisms is being used by a person when he or she reverts from the present level of psychosexual adjustment to a more immature level:

    A. Rationalization

    B. Sublimation

    C. Repression

    D. Regression

96. Which of these statements is *not* relevant to a client with neurosis?

    A. Thought processes may be impaired
    B. Regressive behavior
    C. Impaired judgment
    D. A minimal loss of contact with reality

97. All the following apply to schizophrenia, *except:*

    A. The onset is at middle age
    B. Delusions may be present
    C. Hallucinations may be present
    D. There is a break with reality

Part D

Media

Select the Most Appropriate Answer

1. The proper sequence to follow when making a copper tooling project is:
    A. Tracing design—tooling—filling back of design—mounting—oxidizing—finishing
    B. Tracing design—tooling—filling back of design—oxidizing—finishing—mounting
    C. Tracing design—filling back of design—tooling—mounting—oxidizing—finishing
    D. Tracing design—filling back of design—tooling—oxidizing—finishing—mounting

2. The basic elements needed to operate a puppet show are:
    A. Puppet, theme, script, skit, and stage
    B. Puppeteer, creativity, puppet, script, and stage
    C. Puppet, theme, script, stage, and self-expression
    D. Puppet, theme, marionette, script, and stage

3. When working on a macramé project, how many strands does one need to make a square knot?
    A. Five
    B. Three
    C. Four
    D. Seven

4. A series of square knots form a:
    A. Lark's head
    B. Solomon bar
    C. Half hitch knot
    D. Half knot

5. When working with ceramic tiles one uses grout mixed with water to:
    A. Hold mosaic material to the background
    B. Polish the ceramic tiles
    C. Make a mosaic design
    D. Fill the spaces between the mosaic pieces

6. The type of prehension pattern used while holding a hammer is:

    A. Hook

    B. Cylindrical

    C. Lateral

    D. Three-jaw chuck

7. The type of pinch used while holding a nail is:

    A. Fingertip pinch

    B. Three-point pinch

    C. Key pinch

    D. Palmar pinch

8. The joint action of the wrist while hammering is:

    A. Circumduction

    B. Flexion and extension

    C. Radial and ulnar deviation

    D. Rotation

9. The joint action of the elbow while hammering is:

    A. Rotation

    B. Flexion and extension

    C. Circumduction

    D. Adduction and abduction

10. In order to increase resistance while hammering nails one could:

    A. Use fewer nails

    B. Use harder wood

    C. Use larger nails and a heavier hammer

    D. Both B and C

11. Which of the following activities is not primarily performed in the occupational therapy (OT) department?

    A. Weaving

    B. Splinting

    C. Activities of daily living

    D. Specific gait-training goals

    E. Training on adaptive aids

12. All activities and tasks requiring verbal instructions contain:
    A. Tactile stimuli
    B. Kinesthetic stimuli
    C. Visual stimuli
    D. Auditory stimuli

13. What sensory modalities are involved in the activity of rolling out putty into a coil?
    A. Tactile
    B. Kinesthetic
    C. Visual
    D. All the above

14. The use of the staple gun requires:
    A. Fingertip prehension
    B. Hook grasp
    C. Cylindrical grasp
    D. Lateral prehension

15. The challenge of hand puppetry is capturing the movements of the human body and projecting them through the hands into the puppet. Locomotion movements are mainly made by the:
    A. Shoulder
    B. Arm
    C. Wrist
    D. Thumb

16. The joint action(s) of the elbow when lacing a leather wallet is/are:
    A. Rotation
    B. Circumduction
    C. Adduction and abduction
    D. Flexion and extension

17. The joint action(s) of the shoulder while hammering nails in a woodwork project is/are:
    A. Flexion and extension
    B. Circumduction
    C. Internal and external rotation
    D. Adduction and abduction

18. The most common prehension pattern seen when using the copper tooling stick is:
    A. Fingertip
    B. Palmar tripod (three-jaw chuck)
    C. Lateral
    D. Hook

19. Occupation is the goal-directed use of a person's:
    A. Time
    B. Energy
    C. Interest
    D. All the above

20. The purpose of skiving leather is to:
    A. Reduce thickness
    B. Reduce shrinkage
    C. Align edges of different pieces
    D. Improve the grain of the leather

21. Pieces of leather that will be laced together should be skived to:
    A. Align the lace holes in both pieces
    B. Reduce bulkiness when the pieces are laced
    C. Minimize differences in grain between the pieces
    D. Prevent edges of both pieces from shrinking

22. The function of thonging chisels is to:
    A. Force lace through leather
    B. Cut slits into leather
    C. Groove leather so lacing will be straight
    D. Round corners on pieces of leather

23. A one-pronged thonging chisel should be used when:
    A. Cutting corner slits
    B. Lacing through first and last openings
    C. A single groove is needed
    D. Leather is soft and thin

24. Leather is moistened before it is carved to:
    A.   Shrink it
    B.   Darken it
    C.   Soften it
    D.   Clean it

25. In order to push the ridges of the design template into the moistened leather, one uses:
    A.   A modeling tool with one firm stroke
    B.   A modeling tool with smooth overlapping strokes
    C.   The hand to press the template down slowly
    D.   The hand to press the template down quickly

26. Ripples along the edge of a cut made into leather are caused by:
    A.   A swivel knife with a dull blade
    B.   A swivel knife with a tilted blade
    C.   Leather that is too moist
    D.   Leather that is too dry

27. A thin raised edge along one side of a cut made into leather is caused by:
    A.   Too much pressure on the knife barrel
    B.   Not enough pressure on the knife barrel
    C.   A tilted knife blade
    D.   A dull knife blade

28. In leather carving, the depth of a cut is controlled by:
    A.   Thumb pressure
    B.   Index finger pressure
    C.   The sharpness of the blade
    D.   Barrel adjustment

29. When carving leather, the correct position of the index finger on the swivel knife is on:
    A.   The barrel, next to the second finger
    B.   The barrel, opposite the thumb
    C.   The top of the yoke
    D.   The side of the yoke

30. The manner in which a patient approaches an activity can give the therapist information concerning:

    A. The patient's ability to follow directions
    B. The patient's organizational skills
    C. The patient's religious preference
    D. Both A and B

31. When picking up a greenware mug one should:

    A. Hold it by the rim with one hand
    B. Hold it by the handle
    C. Place both hands around the mug and lift it carefully
    D. It doesn't matter how the mug is held

32. Glazes that fire to a soft dull finish are:

    A. Matte glazes
    B. Majolica gloss glaze
    C. Crackle glaze
    D. None of the above

33. The glazing method that should be used to glaze the inside of hollow pieces such as pitchers, vases, etc. is:

    A. Pouring
    B. Brushing
    C. Spraying
    D. Dipping

34. Glazes should be applied by using:

    A. Five coats
    B. One coat only
    C. Four coats
    D. Two to three coats

35. Pyramids made from clay used as indicators of heat within the kiln are called:

    A. Stilts
    B. Shelf supports
    C. Fire bricks
    D. Pyrometric cones

36. Items needed in stacking the kiln for glaze firing to keep ceramic objects from touching shelves are:

   A. Stilts
   B. Slips
   C. Cones
   D. Pyramids

37. The method of forming clay used in the potter's wheel is called:

   A. Throwing
   B. Slab
   C. Mold
   D. Coil

38. When a client shows interest in making a ceramic piece using the coil method, the therapist must give him or her:

   A. Clay and water
   B. A fettling knife
   C. A and B
   D. A rolling pin

39. Therapeutic activities will be successful when they are:

   A. Relevant to the group
   B. Meaningful and relevant to the clients
   C. Relevant only to the individual
   D. Meaningful to the therapist

40. In general terms, therapeutic activities must be:

   A. Goal oriented
   B. For the patient's enjoyment
   C. Fulfilling for the therapist
   D. Pleasurable for those around the patient

41. When planning a therapeutic craft program for a patient, the therapist should be aware that:

   A. A therapeutic craft program does not need an explanation because the OT profession is in its adulthood
   B. Therapeutic craft programs are often misunderstood by the patient
   C. Therapeutic craft programs are often misunderstood by other health professionals
   D. B and C

42. Within treatment planning, selecting a specific media to be used is based on the:
    A. Skill of the person
    B. Activity analysis and person's learning type
    C. Skill of the therapist
    D. Materials existent in the OT clinic

43. Purposeful activities should be interesting and acceptable to the patient. Also, activities are intended to:
    A. Be fun for the person
    B. Show accomplishment through the end product
    C. Be a diversion from the patient's pathology
    D. Show their relationship to overall rehabilitation goals

44. A slab of plaster, used to dry moist clay or to work on, is called:
    A. Modeling wheel
    B. Bat
    C. Mold
    D. Stilt

45. The most commonly used type of clay is:
    A. Stoneware
    B. Fire clay
    C. Porcelain
    D. Earthenware

46. The type of clay that does not need to be waterproofed when fired is:
    A. Fire clay
    B. Stoneware
    C. Earthenware
    D. Porcelain

47. The dropping of the latch on the electric kiln during firing indicates that the:
    A. Kiln should remain on high for one more hour
    B. Kiln load has reached maturity, and the kiln should be turned off
    C. Fan should be turned on
    D. Fire brick should be removed

48. Clay that has been fired once in the kiln is called:
    A. Leatherhard
    B. Glazeware
    C. Greenware
    D. Bisque

49. The type of clay used for insulating brick, firebrick, and kiln furniture is:
    A. Earthenware
    B. Stoneware
    C. Fire clay
    D. Porcelain

50. The type of clay that does not need firing is termed:
    A. Porcelain
    B. Mexican pottery clay
    C. Leatherhard clay
    D. None of the above

51. When using the mold method in ceramics, the first step is one of the following:
    A. Pouring slip
    B. Centering
    C. Shaping
    D. Removing from the wheel

52. The contraction process of a clay piece as a result of evaporation and expulsion of water during drying and firing is called:
    A. Wedging
    B. Shrinkage
    C. Plasticity
    D. Spraying

53. Activities that may prevent preoccupation are:
    A. Menial tasks such as tearing rags for rugs
    B. Finger painting or punching leather
    C. Stenciling, basketry, or woodworking
    D. Cleaning up the clinic area or other maintenance activities

54. Regressive activities include:

    A. Simple mosaics and sanding wood

    B. Finger painting and copper tooling with template

    C. Therapeutic pottery and clinic maintenance

    D. All the above

55. Activity/activities that would help alleviate guilt is/are:

    A. Floor loom weaving

    B. Printing

    C. Menial tasks

    D. Projects that are gifts for others

    E. Jewelry

    F. C and D

56. Activities that would encourage socialization are:

    A. Paper collage and task groups

    B. Stamping and carving leather

    C. Basketry and stenciling

    D. Sawing wood and metal

57. In woodwork, the function of a plane is to:

    A. Smooth, shape, and level surfaces of wood

    B. Cut angles in wood

    C. Countersink a pilot hole

    D. Decorate surfaces of wood

58. In woodwork, the joint illustrated is called (Figure 2-8):

    A. Lap

    B. Butt

    C. Rabbet

    D. Miter

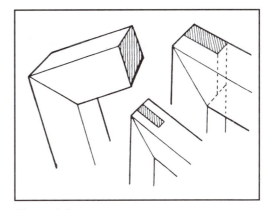

Figure 2-8.

59. The size of grits in sandpaper determines one of the following:
    A. Size
    B. Strength
    C. Cost
    D. Grade

60. Which of the following abrasives is the finest?
    A. Number 1½
    B. Number 3
    C. Number 4/0
    D. Number 8/0

61. The size of a jigsaw is determined by the distance from the upright arm to the:
    A. Tension sleeve
    B. Upper head
    C. Table
    D. Blade

62. A claw hammer is used to:
    A. Hammer all types of nails
    B. Remove claw holders
    C. Remove finishing nails only
    D. Do upholstering work

63. When driving nails one must:
    A. Hold the hammer at the end of the handle
    B. Drill a small hole first when using hardwood
    C. Stagger nails to prevent splitting the wood
    D. Start by pounding the nail with one heavy blow

64. When cutting a project from wood, the saw cut is made:
    A. On the line
    B. Outside the line
    C. Inside the line
    D. It doesn't matter

65. A saw that fits into a frame to cut angles is a:

    A. Rip saw
    B. Hack saw
    C. Coping saw
    D. Miter saw

66. Which of the following requires the user to wear safety goggles?

    A. Table saw
    B. Lathe
    C. Sander
    D. All the above

67. Identify the tool in the picture (Figure 2-9):

    A. Gouge
    B. Bench plane
    C. Sander
    D. Vise

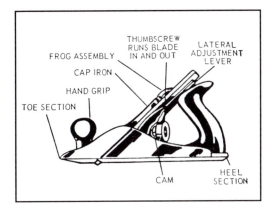

Figure 2-9.

68. The tool in the picture is called (Figure 2-10):

    A. File
    B. Screwdriver
    C. Chisel
    D. Gouge

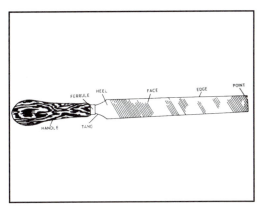

Figure 2-10.

69. The tool in the picture is one of the following (Figure 2-11):

    A. Automatic drill
    B. Ratchet brace
    C. Twist drill
    D. Breast drill

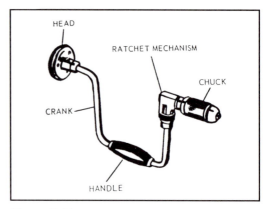

Figure 2-11.

70. The tool in the picture is a(n) (Figure 2-12):

    A. Frame saw
    B. Joint box
    C. Angle saw
    D. Miter box

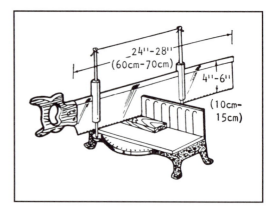

Figure 2-12.

71. Identify the tool in the picture (Figure 2-13):

    A. Ratchet screwdriver
    B. Offset screwdriver
    C. Standard screwdriver
    D. Phillips screwdriver

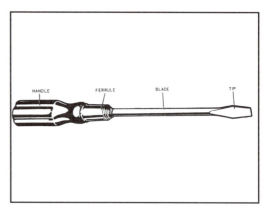

Figure 2-13.

72. Which of the following is the clamp shown in this picture (Figure 2-14)?

    A. Band screw clamp
    B. Bar screw clamp
    C. C-clamp
    D. Corner clamp

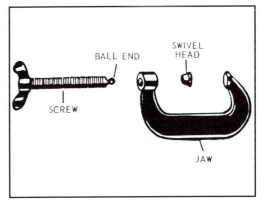

Figure 2-14.

73. In woodwork, the joint illustrated in the picture is called (Figure 2-15):

    A. Mortise-and-tenon
    B. Spline
    C. Dovetail
    D. Dowel

74. In order to drive a finishing nail into top surface wood, one uses a:

    A. Nail set
    B. Ball pien hammer
    C. Depth gauge
    D. Countersink

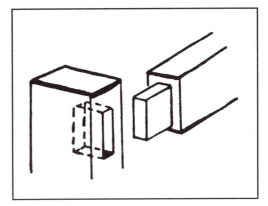

Figure 2-15.

75. Copper tooling is a versatile and inexpensive craft. One of the following is used in this activity:

    A. Chisel
    B. Revolving punch
    C. Liver of sulfur
    D. Mallet

Section II Crossword Puzzle

Physical Dysfunctions—Occupational Therapy Terminology

Across

1. Tuberculosis (abbr.)
2. Xray view (abbr.)
4. Spinal cord dysfunction (abbr.)
6. Therapeutic activity
10. Absence of one or more limbs
12. Gerontic activity (abbr.)
14. Nurse (abbr.)
15. Arm (abbr. reversed)
16. Spoon and fork combination
18. One of the senses
20. Volar
21. Physiatrist (abbr.)
22. Level of upper limb amputation (abbr.)
23. One finger, other than the thumb
29. Sample
30. Thumb
33. Exclamation
37. Little's disease (abbr.)
38. Against
39. Welfare agency (abbr.)
41. Information
43. Feeding utensil
45. Parkinson's disease
49. Twice daily (abbr.)
50. At birth
51. Component of the upper extremity prosthesis (abbr.)
53. Thumb joint (abbr.)
54. Cancer (abbr.)
55. Manual muscle test (abbr.)
56. Opposite of yes

Down

1. Traumatic brain injury (abbr.)
2. Morning (abbr.)
3. Fruit skin
4. Sensory integration (abbr.)
5. Joint immobilization procedure
7. Department in hospital setting (abbr.)
8. Flexor versus extensor
9. Personal identifications (abbr.)
11. Hand muscles with triple action
12. Range of motion (abbr.)
13. Surgery suite (abbr.)
17. Youngster (slang)
19. Caudal
20. Public relations (abbr.)
21. Finger joint (abbr.)
24. Intramuscularly (abbr.)
25. One part of the psyche
26. Connects muscle to bone
27. Medial side of the arm
28. Heart attack (abbr.)
31. Neurological dysfunction (abbr.)
32. Hand brace
33. Carpal bone
34. Being in operation
35. Radiation
36. Multiple sclerosis (abbr.)
40. Afterwards
41. Mother's husband (slang)
42. Surgical removal of adenoids and tonsils (abbr.)
44. Ache
45. Finger joint (abbr.)
46. Like (reversed)
47. The state of Georgia (abbr.)
48. Sick
49. Prefix indicating two
52. Drug addiction (abbr. reversed)

Answer Key

Section II
Theory—Part A

Pediatrics

1. A. Athetoid. **2.** D. Grady. **3.** A. Motor cortex. **4.** D. A mixture of different approaches. **5.** B. Give detailed verbal instructions. **6.** C. Circle. **7.** E. Both A) To promote motor skills and C) To elicit cooperative play attitudes. **8.** D. Both A) Nurturing and C) Structured. **9.** D. "Snake-like" movements **10.** B. "Sway-back."

11. E. Both A) Cephalocaudal and D) Proximal to distal. **12.** A. Triangle **13.** B. Unilateral. **14.** C. Hands and forearms. **15.** C. Three-dimensional objects. **16.** B. Left. **17.** B. By school age. **18.** C. Ayres. **19.** A. Chromosomal abnormality. **20.** C. Self-devaluation.

21. C. Motor planning. **22.** C. Too rapidly. **23.** B. An exaggerated anterior convexity of the spine. **24.** A. Progressive degeneration of voluntary musculature. **25.** A. Sensory reception of stimuli. **26.** C. Inability of self-expression through speech. **27.** B. Ability to know how an object is turned. **28.** C. Repetition of what is said but the meaning is not associated with the words. **29.** C. Ability of the observer to perceive the position of two or more objects in relation to himself or herself and to each other. **30.** B. Ability to follow a moving object with the eyes.

31. A. Intense withdrawal. **32.** B. Sensory and/or motor deficits. **33.** C. Only toes touch the floor. **34.** A. Paralysis of one limb. **35.** C. A genetic abnormality. **36.** B. Exploratory. **37.** D. All the above. **38.** C. Higher than the well population. **39.** A. Paraplegia. **40.** B. Spasticity of muscles.

41. A. Bowel reaches maturity before the bladder. **42.** D. Both A) Eye poking and C) A characteristic of the visually impaired. **43.** D. All the above. **44.** C. A circle. **45.** B. Acalculia. **46.** D. Motor development occurs in the caudal–cephalad direction. **47.** D. All the above. **48.** A. Inability to speak clearly because of weakness of the muscles of phonation. **49.** B. Neurodevelopmental treatment. **50.** D. Both B) Withdrawal reflexes and C) Flexion reflexes.

51. A. Clumsiness. **52.** A. Fingertip pads. **53.** D. Bladder management. **54.** B. Volar area of the hand on the ulnar side. **55.** C. Developmental delay. **56.** B. The central nervous system is still immature and primitive patterns are not strongly developed. **57.** B. A child acquires higher functions by the modification of lower level responses. **58.** C. Vestibular. **59.** D. Proprioception. **60.** A. Kinesthesia.

61. D. Physical pain. **62.** C. Tactile and vestibular. **63.** B. Verbalization. **64.** C. Carl Rogers. **65.** C. Association, accommodation, assimilation, and differentiation. **66.** A. Echolalia. **67.** C. Lack of order. **68.** D. Both A) Form perception and position in space and C) Depth perception and figure/ground perception. **69.** C. Sensorimotor. **70.** D. Both B) Upper motor neuron and C) Lower motor neuron.

71. C. Parallel play. **72.** D. High. **73.** C. Bow legs. **74.** C. Define problems. **75.** C. Mobility mechanism. **76.** D. High intellectual ability. **77.** A. Rolling. **78.** D. Juvenile rheumatoid arthritis. **79.** B. In childhood. **80.** B. Influenza. **81.** D. Increased interaction with peers.

Part B

Physical Dysfunction

1. B. Denial. **2.** A. Sliding door with top and bottom runners. **3.** B. Pressure mat door. **4.** D. All the above. **5.** B. Refrigerator, sink, and cooking facilities. **6.** B. More life space than the average person. **7.** D. Both B) One cannot understand verbal directions and C) One cannot understand written directions. **8.** E. Answers A) Ability to read, C) Ability to listen, and D) Ability to speak. **9.** C. Carcinoma. **10.** B. Cartilage.

11. C. Drop wrist. **12.** E. All the above. **13.** B. No moving parts. **14.** D. Compound. **15.** D. Both A) Sustained pull and B) Pull in the proper direction to maintain the alignment of the fragments. **16.** C. Simple. **17.** C. Rocker knife. **18.** B. The area downward from the trunk. **19.** C. The angles of joints. **20.** B. Baltimore treatment equipment.

21. D. Both B) Exercise the free joints as much as possible and C) Exercise adjacent joints to the cast. **22.** B. Physical medicine modality. **23.** C. One side of the body (right or left). **24.** B. To keep the shoulder free of contractures. **25.** D. A bone that fractures incompletely. **26.** C. Hematoma. **27.** B. Proximal interphalangeals. **28.** C. Standing rather than sitting when ironing. **29.** D. Thumb opposition. **30.** D. Ankylosing spondylitis.

31. A. A first-degree burn. **32.** A. Rheumatoid arthritis. **33.** D. Thrombosis. **34.** B. Gouty arthritis. **35.** D. Passive ROM during the acute stage. **36.** A. Young adulthood. **37.** B. Late adulthood. **38.** D. All the above. **39.** B. Hypotonicity of the muscles. **40.** A. Prevention of decubitus.

41. E. All the above. **42.** A. Tenodesis hand splint. **43.** B. Hypertonicity of muscles. **44.** C. Wrist joint. **45.** C. There is destruction of the entire thickness of the skin. **46.** A. Flaccid. **47.** D. Scanned speech. **48.** B. Active motion. **49.** B. Shoulder internally rotated and adducted; elbow, wrist, and fingers flexed. **50.** C. "Frozen shoulder."

51. A. External rotation. **52.** C. A speech pathologist. **53.** C. Shoulder-hand syndrome. **54.** D. Ischemia. **55.** D. All the above. **56.** A. Shoulder flexion. **57.** D. Anterior horn cells. **58.** B. Sitting with good positioning patterns close to a table. **59.** A. 32 in. **60.** A. Functional position.

61. A. Resist flexion in uninvolved upper extremity. **62.** A. Quick motor response. **63.** C. A person with good visual acuity who cannot match shapes or objects. **64.** A. Muscle strength. **65.** A. It prevents hyperextension of the metacarpophalangeal joints (MCPJs). **66.** B. Shoulder and elbow muscles. **67.** D. Keep good positioning. **68.** A. Isotonic assistive. **69.** E. All the above. **70.** A. Stupor.

71. C. Neglect of one extremity. **72.** C. Boutonniere. **73.** C. Elderly women. **74.** D. Soft tissue strain. **75.** B. Tremors, rigidity, and slowness of movement. **76.** A. Bradykinesia. **77.** A. Orthoplast, polyform, and aquaplast. **78.** C. 15 to 29 years old. **79.** C. III. **80.** C. Bilateral symmetrical.

81. B. Passive. **82.** D. Degree of the patient's motivation. **83.** B. Two thirds of the forearm. **84.** A. Elevating. **85.** D. Sensitive enough to detect minor changes. **86.** C. The biceps, the three portions of the trapezius, and serratus anterior. **87.** B. Resting tremors. **88.** B. The inability to adduct the wrist. **89.** D. All the above. **90.** D. C5 to C6.

91. C. A terminal device. **92.** D. Remissions and exacerbations. **93.** D. Work adjustment programs. **94.** D. Swan neck. **95.** D. Both A) Right hemiparesia and C) Left hemiparesia. **96.** E. Both B) Shortness of breath and D) Chest pain or pressure. **97.** D. Dorsiflexion. **98.** B. Hip internal rotation, abduction and extension, knee extension, ankle plantar flexion and inversion, and toes flexion. **99.** B. 29½ in. **100.** B. Dynamometer.

101. A. Pinch gauge. **102.** D. Dynamometer. **103.** C. Goniometer. **104.** B. Cock-up hand splint. **105.** A. Resting pan hand splint. **106.** D. Tenodesis hand splint. **107.** C. Opponens hand splint. **108.** C. Heberden's nodes. **109.** A. Sudden onset. **110.** D. Difficulty in swallowing.

111. D. Surgical sectioning of a bone. **112.** C. An operation to restore mobility to a stiffened joint. **113.** D. Osteosarcoma. **114.** A. Median nerve. **115.** C. Ectomy. **116.** A. Myectomy. **117.** C. Endurance increases. **118.** B. Scleroderma. **119.** C. It is characterized by joint wear and tear.

Part C

Psychosocial Dysfunction

1. D. Denial—anger—bargaining—depression—acceptance. **2.** C. Loss of appetite. **3.** C. Conversion reaction. **4.** A. Docile. **5.** C. Verbal recognition of the patient's feelings. **6.** C. Unstructured activities. **7.** D. A) A clonic phase and B) A tonic phase. **8.** D. All of the above. **9.** E. All the above. **10.** B. Delusion.

11. C. Hallucinations. **12.** A. Catatonic. **13.** B. Anal. **14.** A. Release therapy. **15.** C. A time of dependency. **16.** A. Reactive depression. **17.** C. Psychosis. **18.** B. Perception. **19.** D. Depersonalization. **20.** B. Ethics, self-criticism.

21. A. Depression. **22.** C. Mania. **23.** B. Illusion. **24.** B. Affective domain. **25.** A. Echolalia. **26.** D. Conduct disorders. **27.** C. Processing of sensory information so an individual can act in the environment. **28.** A. The environment is considered objectively. **29.** B. A task group. **30.** D. Intermember similarities.

31. A. When one engages in interaction with another. **32.** C. Physiological. **33.** D. All the above. **34.** C. Interpreting. **35.** D. Your feelings are unimportant. **36.** C. Condescending attitude. **37.** B. Conflict. **38.** C. Safety. **39.** E. All the above. **40.** C. One's inner tensions are expressed symbolically and disguised.

41. B. Thinking well of oneself. **42.** D. Thought. **43.** E. Both A) Social comparison and D) Reflected appraisal. **44.** C. Spiritual, intellectual, organic. **45.** D. Maladaptive behavior. **46.** B. Instead of discussing a problem, the person pretends it doesn't exist. **47.** C. Memory. **48.** C. Operates on the "reality principle." **49.** B. Ability to relate to others. **50.** B. The person's enjoyment interests.

51. D. Ambivalence. **52.** C. A deficient ability to process information internally. **53.** A. Using avoidance, denial, and repudiation. **54.** C. Reaction formation. **55.** A. Complete and sudden loss of consciousness. **56.** C. An emotional reliving of stressful situations. **57.** A. Metabolic imbalances. **58.** B. Delusion. **59.** A. Negativism. **60.** D. Selective.

61. A. Paranoid. **62.** C. Intellectual function. **63.** C. Conversion reaction. **64.** A. Irrational fears. **65.** B. Perserveration. **66.** B. Has difficulty maintaining socially acceptable behavior. **67.** C. Freud. **68.** C. Concern arises regarding physical differences between boys and girls. **69.** D. Sudden withdrawal of alcohol from a chronic alcoholic. **70.** B. Memory.

71. B. The therapist's attitudes toward the patient. **72.** C. Antianxiety. **73.** C. Reality therapy. **74.** C. American Psychiatric Association. **75.** A. Antipsychotic agent. **76.** D. Affect. **77.** C. Self-admiration. **78.** B. Increased social interests. **79.** A. Inadequate job skills. **80.** C. Indecisiveness.

81. D. Paranoia. **82.** A. Acrophobia. **83.** A. Projection. **84.** B. Perfectionism. **85.** D. Denial. **86.** A. Conversion reaction. **87.** C. Makes voluntary decisions. **88.** B. Basic instinctual drives. **89.** A. Anal. **90.** A. Depression.

91. C. Overtly displaying aggression. **92.** B. Claustrophobia. **93.** C. A conversion reaction. **94.** C. The patient retains reality-testing functions. **95.** D. Regression. **96.** B. Regressive behavior. **97.** A. The onset is at middle age.

Part D

Media

1. B. Tracing design—tooling—filling back of design—oxidizing—finishing—mounting. **2.** A. Puppet, theme, script, skit, and stage. **3.** C. Four. **4.** B. Solomon bar. **5.** D. Fill the spaces between the mosaic pieces. **6.** B. Cylindrical. **7.** A. Fingertip pinch. **8.** C. Radial and ulnar deviation. **9.** B. Flexion and extension. **10.** D. Both B) Use harder wood and C) Use larger nails and a heavier hammer.

11. D. Specific gait-training goals. **12.** D. Auditory stimuli. **13.** D. All the above. **14.** C. Cylindrical grasp. **15.** A. Shoulder. **16.** D. Flexion and extension. **17.** A. Flexion and extension. **18.** B. Palmar tripod (three-jaw chuck) **19.** D. All the above. **20.** A. Reduce thickness.

21. B. Reduce bulkiness when the pieces are laced. **22.** B. Cut slits into leather. **23.** A. Cutting corner slits. **24.** C. Soften it. **25.** B. A modeling tool with smooth overlapping strokes. **26.** A. A swivel knife with a dull blade. **27.** C. A tilted knife blade. **28.** B. Index finger pressure. **29.** C. The top of the yoke. **30.** D. Both A) The patient's ability to follow directions and B) The patient's organizational skills.

31. C. Place both hands around the mug and lift it carefully. **32.** A. Matte glazes. **33.** A. Pouring. **34.** D. Two to three coats. **35.** D. Pyrometric cones. **36.** A. Stilts. **37.** A. Throwing. **38.** C. Both A) Clay and water and B) A fettling knife. **39.** B. Meaningful and relevant to the clients. **40.** A. Goal oriented.

41. D. Both B) Therapeutic craft programs are often misunderstood by the patient and C) Therapeutic craft programs are often misunderstood by other health professionals. **42.** B. Activity analysis and person's learning type. **43.** D. Show their relationship to overall rehabilitation goals. **44.** B. Bat. **45.** D. Earthenware. **46.** B. Stoneware. **47.** B. Kiln load has reached maturity, and the kiln should be turned off. **48.** D. Bisque. **49.** C. Fire clay. **50.** B. Mexican pottery clay.

51. A. Pouring slip. **52.** B. Shrinkage. **53.** C. Stenciling, basketry, or woodworking. **54.** D. All the above. **55.** F. Both C) Menial tasks and D) Projects that are gifts for others. **56.** A. Paper collage and task groups. **57.** A. Smooth, shape, and level surfaces of wood. **58.** D. Miter. **59.** D. Grade. **60.** D. Number 8/0.

61. D. Blade. **62.** A. Hammer all types of nails. **63.** B. Drill a small hole first when using hardwood. **64.** B. Outside the line. **65.** D. Miter saw. **66.** D. All the above. **67.** B. Bench plane. **68.** A. File. **69.** B. Ratchet brace. **70.** D. Miter box.

71. C. Standard screwdriver. **72.** C. C-clamp. **73.** A. Mortise-and-tenon. **74.** A. Nail set. **75.** C. Liver of sulfur.

Key

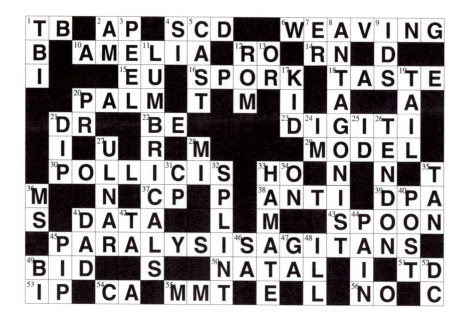

Across

1. TB
2. AP (Anterior and Posterior)
4. SCD
6. Weaving
10. Amelia
12. RO (Reality Orientation)
14. RN (Registered Nurse)
15. EU (Upper Extremity)
16. Spork
18. Taste
20. Palm
21. DR (Doctor)
22. BE (Below Elbow)
23. Digiti
29. Model
30. Pollicis
33. HO
37. CP (Cerebral Palsy)
38. Anti
39. DPA (Department of Public Assistance)
41. Data
43. Spoon
45. Paralysis agitans

49. BID
50. Natal
51. TD (Terminal Device)
53. IP (Inter Phalangeal)
54. CA
55. MMT
56. No

Down

1. TBI
2. AM
3. Peel
4. SI
5. Cast
7. ER (Emergency Room)
8. Antagonist
9. IDs
11. Lumbricals
12. ROM
13. OR (Operating Room)
17. Kid
19. Tail
20. PR
21. DIP (Distal Interphalangeal)

24. IM
25. Id
26. Tendon
27. Ulnar
28. MI (Miocardial Infarct)
31. CP (Cerebral Palsy)
32. Splint
33. Hamate
34. On
35. Tan
36. MS
40. Post
41. Dad
42. TA (Tonsilectomy and Adenoidectomy)
44. Pain
45. PIP (Proximal Interphalangeal)
46. Sa
47. GA
48. Ill
49. Bi
52. DC (Chemical Dependency)

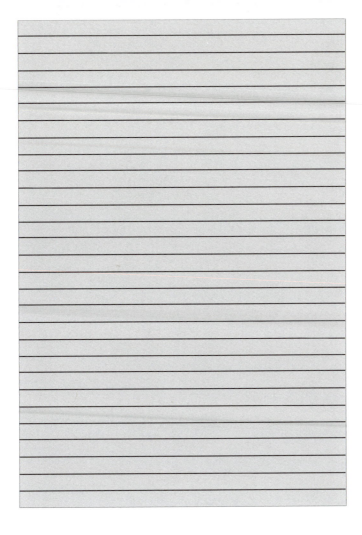

SECTION III

Administration and Management

Select the Most Appropriate Answer

1. The entry level certified occupational therapy assistant (COTA) has sufficient knowledge to perform:
   A. Regular evaluations
   B. Activities of daily living evaluations
   C. Hemiplegic evaluations
   D. All the above

2. When the therapist writes progress notes, he or she may use the "SOAP" method. What does the initial "A" stand for?
   A. Acute symptoms
   B. Action
   C. Artifacts
   D. Assessment

3. When the therapist writes progress notes, he or she may use the "SOAP" method. What does the initial "S" stand for?
   A. Social history
   B. Symptoms
   C. Subjective
   D. Sequelae

4. Funding for occupational therapy (OT) services rendered is obtained from:
   A. The state government
   B. Private insurance companies
   C. The federal government
   D. Direct patient payment
   E. All the above

5. The term of office of the representative assembly is:

    A. 6 months

    B. 5 years

    C. 2 years

    D. 3 years

6. The first national certification examination for COTAs was administered in:

    A. 1980

    B. 1975

    C. 1970

    D. 1977

7. A telephone call is received from an attorney asking about a specific patient's status; the COTA should:

    A. Hang up the telephone

    B. Allow the patient to handle the situation by himself or herself

    C. Give the attorney the requested information

    D. Tell the attorney that this type of information is confidential

8. A physical medicine and rehabilitation department includes:

    A. OT

    B. Physical therapy

    C. Speech therapy

    D. All the above

    E. A and B only

9. In a problem oriented medical record, a progress note states, "patient reaches over head to comb her hair and is able to dress without assistance." This statement should be recorded under which of the following:

    A. Treatment plan

    B. Subjective information

    C. Objective data

    D. Assessment

10. When a COTA is assisting in the development of a new OT service in a home health program, the first step should be:

    A. Establishing program goals
    B. Completing a needs assessment
    C. Training volunteers
    D. Identifying reimbursement sources

11. Requests for OT services may come from the:

    A. Physician
    B. Nursing department
    C. Physical therapist
    D. Teachers
    E. All the above

12. The telephone number of the OT national office is: 1-800-:

    A. THE-AOTA
    B. PAY-AOTA
    C. SAY-AOTA
    D. FOR-AOTA

13. Which of the following publications are distributed by the American Occupational Therapy Association (AOTA)?

    A. *American Journal of Occupational Therapy (AJOT)*
    B. *OT Week*®
    C. *OT Forum*
    D. A, B, and C
    E. A and B

14. The representative assembly is the:

    A. Legislative element of the AOTA
    B. Executive body of the AOTA
    C. Policy making component of the AOTA
    D. A and C

15. Within patient documentation, the therapist should:

    A. Use formal language
    B. Use medical terminology appropriately
    C. Write in the third person
    D. All the above

16. Within OT, the term "consultation" means:
    A. To plan, supervise, and direct others
    B. To provide training and information
    C. To implement a program
    D. To plan a treatment program

17. When did the AOTA begin a program of approval of educational programs for occupational therapy assistants (OTAs)?
    A. 1959
    B. 1967
    C. 1935
    D. 1945

18. The function of the accreditation committee is the approval of one of the following:
    A. Certification of the COTA
    B. Registration of the registered occupational therapist (OTR)
    C. OT standards of practice
    D. OT educational programs
    E. Principles of OT ethics

19. The executive director of the AOTA is:
    A. The manager of the representative assembly
    B. Elected by the AOTA membership
    C. Employed by the national association
    D. The manager of the world federation of occupational therapy

20. An AOTA member is considered to be in good standing when he or she:
    A. Writes articles for the *AJOT* or *Advance for Occupational Therapists*™
    B. Pays his or her yearly national fee
    C. Passes the national certification examination
    D. Belongs to a particular special interest group

21. Formal research in OT is:
    A. Contraindicated
    B. Well established
    C. In its beginning
    D. Necessary to the growth of the profession
    E. C and D
    F. B and D

22. The certification examination for the COTA is administered by:

    A. The AOTA
    B. The individual state association
    C. The National Board of Certification in Occupational Therapy, Inc. (NBCOT)
    D. The licensure board

23. The occupational therapist should actively participate periodically in continuing education programs because:

    A. It is a licensure requirement
    B. Of promotion purposes
    C. OT information is constantly increasing/changing
    D. It is required by the American Medical Association (AMA)
    E. It is required by the AOTA

24. Patient documentation is necessary for:

    A. Communication within team members
    B. Legal implications
    C. Evaluation of the effectiveness of OT services
    D. Research purposes
    E. All the above
    F. A and C

25. Certification and licensure for COTAs are:

    A. Granted by a nongovernmental agency (certification) and a governmental agency (licensure)
    B. The same thing
    C. Both granted by a state agency
    D. Both granted by a national agency

26. The principles of OT ethics are to be used:

    A. By the state OT association
    B. By the institutions that have OT educational programs
    C. Primarily within the OT profession
    D. By the national government
    E. By the state government

27. According to the entry-level COTA role delineations developed by the AOTA, COTAs are allowed to perform OT services only under the supervision of the:

    A. Physical therapist
    B. Speech pathologist
    C. Nursing director
    D. OTR

28. One of the methods of OT service delivery is direct service, which means:

    A. The therapist does not have hands-on contact with the patient
    B. The face-to-face relationship between therapist and patient
    C. The focus on prevention
    D. The occupational therapist provides treatment to children who are under the primary care of other agencies

29. Patients' records should be:

    A. Clear
    B. Concise
    C. Accurate
    D. All the above

30. Occupational performance includes, among other elements:

    A. Self-care
    B. Work
    C. Play
    D. All the above

31. Performance components are which of the following:

    A. Hobbies
    B. Leisure/play
    C. Motor and social functioning
    D. Life space

32. When the physician refers a patient to OT, he or she needs to indicate the:

    A. Modalities to be used
    B. Length of treatment time
    C. Objective of the treatment
    D. Necessary adaptive equipment

33. The members of the AOTA who have the right to vote for the national officers are:

    A. OT students
    B. COTAs
    C. OTRs
    D. B and C
    E. All the above

34. Annual fees paid by the AOTA membership are determined by the:

    A. Executive board
    B. President of the association
    C. Representative assembly
    D. American Occupational Therapy Foundation (AOTF)
    E. NBCOT

35. In a department of OT, the most important factor to take into consideration in determining the number of OT staff is:

    A. Type of setting
    B. Size of the institution
    C. Severity of diagnosis
    D. Patient load requirements

36. Membership of the AOTA include:

    A. OTRs
    B. OT students
    C. COTAs
    D. All the above
    E. Only A and C

37. The colors of the OT insignia are:

    A. White and blue
    B. Yellow and red
    C. White, red, and blue
    D. White and red

38. The president of the AOTA is elected by the membership for a term of:

    A. 3 years
    B. 5 years
    C. 2 years
    D. 6 years

39. The evaluation process of a patient follows which of the following sequences:
    A. Screening—comprehensive evaluation—data analysis—treatment plan
    B. Screening—data analysis—treatment plan—comprehensive evaluation
    C. Screening—comprehensive evaluation—treatment plan—data analysis
    D. Screening—data analysis—comprehensive evaluation—treatment plan

40. An OTA student is doing Fieldwork II in a physical dysfunctions setting. The student has a question concerning the implementation of the treatment plan on one of his or her patients. The student should contact:
    A. Another OT student
    B. The physician
    C. The immediate supervisor
    D. The fieldwork coordinator

41. The AOTA offers a number of benefits to the membership. They include one of the following:
    A. The monthly *AJOT*
    B. Providing membership in a specific state
    C. Licensure
    D. The right to vote for officers at the state association

42. What do the initials "DRG" stand for?
    A. Diagnostic ruled groups
    B. Diagnostic related groups
    C. Disease related groups
    D. Diagnostic related generations

43. In a problem oriented medical record, a progress note reads: "patient complains of low back pain when in sitting..." Where does this quote belong?
    A. Assessment
    B. Objective information
    C. Subjective data
    D. Plan

44. In a problem oriented medical record, the short- and long-term goals should be included in:
    A. Plan
    B. Subjective data
    C. Assessment
    D. Objective information

45. In order for the OTA to become certified, he or she must take the certification exam which is:

   A. The same as the exam offered to OTRs
   B. Different from the OTR's exam
   C. The same as the exam for COTAs, but the passing score is lower
   D. The same as the exam for COTAs, but more time is allotted to complete it

46. Every OT educational program must follow certain guidelines called "essentials" developed by the AOTA. These essentials are:

   A. The same for COTAs and OTRs
   B. The same for OTRs and registered physical therapists
   C. The same for aides and COTAs
   D. Different for OTRs and COTAs

47. One of the primary functions of the AOTF is:

   A. Developing scholarships for OT students
   B. Electing AOTA officers
   C. Representing the AOTA in foreign countries
   D. Developing certification exams

48. Occupational therapists may refer patients to:

   A. Any agency approved by his or her own facility
   B. Any other setting or professional
   C. Physical therapists
   D. Other OTRs only

49. One of the methods of patient documentation is the problem oriented record. This specific way of recording progress notes is called:

   A. Occupational therapy standard client care record (OTSCCR)
   B. Sequential operating progress report (SOPR)
   C. Subjective objective assessment plan (SOAP)
   D. Problem oriented report record (PORR)

50. Professionals working in healthcare facilities must follow a code of ethics. Its main purpose is to describe the relationship amongst the clinician, the client, and:

   A. The AMA
   B. The institution
   C. The society
   D. The immediate OT department

51. According to the AOTA role delineations, which of the following is *not* appropriate for an entry-level COTA?

    A. Participation in educational inservices
    B. Coordination of programs
    C. Assistance in treatment planning
    D. Performance of activity analysis

52. The initials PSRO stand for:

    A. Professional standards rules organization
    B. Professional statements review organization
    C. Professional standards review organization
    D. Periodic statements review organization

53. Acquisition of data by the therapist prior to the assessment of a child:

    A. Is not necessary
    B. Is the institution's procedure
    C. Is the therapist's own procedure
    D. Has its advantages and disadvantages

54. A 7-year-old boy is referred to OT to improve social functioning. What is the most useful data about the child's current level of social functioning?

    A. The speech pathologist's evaluation
    B. The pediatrician's physical examination report
    C. The school's report on the child's behavior
    D. The psychologist's report on the child's intellectual ability

55. The SOAP type of progress notes are:

    A. Unstructured
    B. Problem solving
    C. Too lengthy
    D. An uncommon form of note writing

56. The best method to be used by a COTA in patient documentation is to:

    A. Report periodically to the nursing supervisor
    B. Record only as soon as progress occurs
    C. Ask the patient to keep a log of his or her own performance
    D. Routinely summarize the patient's performance in the medical record
    E. Report to the physician

57. What do the initials POMR stand for?

    A. Public orientation medical record
    B. Perform official medical record
    C. Provide oriented medical report
    D. Problem oriented medical record

58. When writing SOAP notes, the COTA must follow a specific sequence dictated by the initials SOAP. In this type of documentation, short-term goals should be stated:

    A. After long-term goals
    B. Before long-term goals
    C. At the same time as long-term goals
    D. It doesn't matter

59. The earliest that the OT assistant is eligible to apply for state licensure is:

    A. When academic course work has been concluded
    B. As soon as Fieldwork II is finished
    C. When the certification exam is over with
    D. As soon as the certification exam results have been received

60. The certification exam that is conducted by the NBCOT can be taken:

    A. When course work has been concluded
    B. When the applicant has applied for state licensure
    C. As soon as the applicant is officially licensed
    D. After the successful completion of Fieldwork II

61. The Omnibus Budget Reconciliation Act is a set of federal regulations governing the care of residents in long-care facilities. This act notes that documentation of resident's goals be stated concisely, following the "MORE" outline. These four initials stand for:

    A. Measurable, obscure, radical, and effective
    B. Measurable, obvious, random, and elective
    C. Measurable, observable, realistic, and explicit
    D. Measurable, occasional, realistic, and evident

62. What do the initials OSHA stand for?

    A. Oregon State Health Alliance
    B. Occupational Safety and Health Administration
    C. Orientation to Schematic Hereditary Abnormalities
    D. Organizational Services for Hospital Awareness

63. The initials PAM stand for?

    A. Public Awareness Model
    B. Psychometric Aptitude Methodology
    C. Physical Agent Modality
    D. Physiological Ability Maneuver

64. What does HMO stand for?

    A. Health Maintenance Organization
    B. Healing Malformed Opening
    C. Healthy Managerial Organization
    D. Heart Malignancy Operation

65. During the OT process, it is important that the therapist does not "overhelp" the patient because this:

    A. Increases the patient's dependency
    B. Decreases the patient's dependency
    C. Increases the patient's independence
    D. Increases the patient's self-sufficiency

66. A mentor is an advisor who, within his or her wisdom, performs the following, *except*:

    A. Advises the student as needed
    B. Learns from the advisor/advisee relationship
    C. Teaches the student
    D. Makes all the major decisions for the student

67. A COTA working in a rehabilitation hospital setting has, among others, the following specific functions *except*:

    A. Awareness of emergency and safety procedures
    B. Identification of environmental hazards
    C. Performance of hand evaluations
    D. Maintenance of equipment and supplies

68. A good healthcare program is on everyone's mind, and as such, OT is one of its elements. The funding for OT services is largely obtained from the following agencies, *except*:

    A. The state government
    B. Private insurance companies
    C. The federal government
    D. Charitable organizations

69. Outpatient OT services are reimbursed by Medicare part B when:
    A. A specific written plan is followed
    B. Ordered by the physical therapist
    C. Ordered by the quality assurance team
    D. The patient demands it

70. A client who is receiving OT services should:
    A. Assume that the insurance provides coverage
    B. Check with his or her own insurance policy
    C. Pay his or her own bill
    D. Expect the state government to pay

71. A 66-year-old man who is bedridden is going home and needs adaptive equipment and medical follow up. Medicare part B will partially reimburse for:
    A. A trapeze bar
    B. Prescribed medications
    C. Doctor's office visits
    D. OT services only

72. All of the following are third-party payers that provide coverage for OT services rendered, *except:*
    A. Blue Cross–Blue Shield
    B. Medicare
    C. Medical assistance (Medicaid)
    D. Red Cross

Trivia Questions

73. The first educational program for OT assistants was begun in the 1960s in:
    A. Milwaukee, Wisconsin
    B. Cresson, Pennsylvania
    C. St. Louis, Missouri
    D. Rockville, Maryland

74. The first master's degree program for OTs was begun at this university:
    A. University of Pennsylvania
    B. University of Toronto
    C. San Jose State University
    D. University of Southern California

75. The beginning salary of an OTR in 1957 was:
    A. $2,000.00 to $4,460.00
    B. $3,328.00 to $3,600.00
    C. $4,295.00 to $6,220.00
    D. $4,000.00 to $6,500.00

Section III Crossword Puzzle

Management Skills—Occupational Therapy Terminology

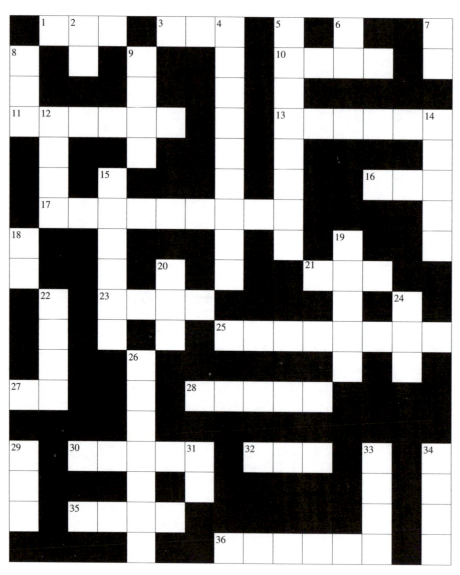

Across

1. Nursing home area in which residents require skilled care (abbr.)

3. Activities of daily living (abbr.)

10. Professional organization that obtains grants and scholarships for occupational therapy students and professionals (abbr.)

11. OT student organization (abbr.)

13. Professional organization (abbr.)

16. Health maintenance organization (reversed abbr.)

17. Method for carrying out policy

21. Professional body involved with issues on education (abbr.)

23. Postsecondary accreditation organization (abbr.)

25. Third-party payer agency

27. Legislative and policy making body of our professional organization (abbr.)

28. Publisher of this book

30. National accreditation agency (abbr.)

32. Nursing home area in which residents do not require skilled care (abbr.)

35. OT student publication (abbr.)

36. Management item without which equipment and supplies cannot be purchased

Down

2. Not applicable (abbr.)

4. It is obtained after one successfully passes the certification exam

5. Budget's biggest item (plural)

6. Member of the rehabilitation team, other than OT (abbr.)

7. Upper extremity amputation level (abbr.)

8. Person who just completed the associate degree in OT (abbr.)

9. Professional organization of the state of Pennsylvania (abbr.)

12. Patient/client documentation method (abbr.)

14. Accreditation body inherent to health professionals (abbr.)

15. It describes how objectives can be met

18. Employment advertisement

19. Former name of the National accreditation board (abbr.)

20. Cardiopulmonary resuscitation (abbr.)

22. Our national professional organization (abbr.)

24. Categorization of different diagnoses (abbr.)

26. Free telephone number used by OT membership

29. National medical organization (abbr.)

31. Member of the rehabilitation team (abbr.)

33. Monthly OT magazine (abbr.)

34. International professional organization (abbr.)

Answer Key

Section III

Administration and Management

1. B. Activities of daily living evaluations. **2.** D. Assessment. **3.** C. Subjective. **4.** E. All the above. **5.** D. 3 years. **6.** D. 1977. **7.** D. Tell the attorney that this type of information is confidential. **8.** D. All the above. **9.** C. Objective data. **10.** B. Completing a needs assessment.

11. E. All the above. **12.** C. SAY-AOTA. **13.** E. Both A) *American Journal of Occupational Therapy* (*AJOT*) and B) *OT Week*®. **14.** D. Both A) Legislative element of the AOTA and C) Policy making component of the AOTA. **15.** D. All the above. **16.** B. To provide training and information. **17.** A. 1959. **18.** D. OT educational programs. **19.** C. Employed by the national association. **20.** B. Pays his or her yearly national fee.

21. E. Both C) In its beginning and D) Necessary to the growth of the profession. **22.** C. The National Board of Certification in Occupational Therapy, Inc. (NBCOT). **23.** C. OT information is constantly increasing/changing. **24.** E. All the above. **25.** A. Granted by a nongovernmental agency (certification) and a governmental agency (licensure). **26.** C. Primarily within the OT profession. **27.** D. OTR. **28.** B. The face-to-face relationship between therapist and patient. **29.** D. All the above. **30.** D. All the above.

31. C. Motor and social functioning. **32.** C. Objective of the treatment. **33.** D. Both B) COTAs and C) OTRs. **34.** C. Representative assembly. **35.** D. Patient load requirements. **36.** D. All the above. **37.** C. White, red, and blue. **38.** A. 3 years. **39.** A. Screening—comprehensive evaluation—data analysis—treatment plan. **40.** C. The immediate supervisor.

41. A. The monthly *AJOT*. **42.** B. Diagnostic related groups. **43.** C. Subjective data. **44.** C. Assessment. **45.** B. Different from the OTR's exam. **46.** D. Different for OTRs and COTAs. **47.** A. Developing scholarships for OT students. **48.** B. Any other setting or professional. **49.** C. Subjective objective assessment plan (SOAP). **50.** C. The society.

51. B. Coordination of programs. **52.** C. Professional standards review organization. **53.** D. Has its advantages and disadvantages. **54.** C. The school's report on the child's behavior. **55.** B. Problem solving. **56.** D. Routinely summarize the patient's performance in the medical record. **57.** D. Problem oriented medical record. **58.** A. After long-term goals. **59.** B. As soon as Fieldwork II is finished. **60.** D. After the successful completion of Fieldwork II.

61. C. Measurable, observable, realistic, and explicit. **62.** B. Occupational Safety and Health Administration. **63.** C. Physical Agent Modality. **64.** A. Health Maintenance Organization. **65.** A. Increases the patient's dependency. **66.** D. Makes all the major decisions for the student. **67.** C. Performance of hand evaluations. **68.** D. Charitable organizations. **69.** A. A specific written plan is followed. **70.** B. Check with his or her own insurance policy.

71. A. A trapeze bar. **72.** D. Red Cross. **73.** B. Cresson, Pennsylvania. **74.** D. University of Southern California. **75.** B. $3,328.00 to $3,600.00.

Key

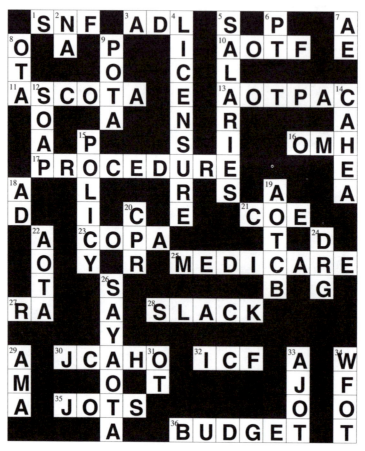

Across

1. SNF (Skilled Nursing Facility)
3. ADL
10. AOTF (American Occupational Therapy Foundation)
11. ASCOTA (American Student Committee of Occupational Therapy)
13. AOTPAC (American Occupational Therapy Political Action Committee)
16. OMH
17. Procedure
21. COE (Commission on Education)
23. COPA (Council on Postsecondary Accreditation)
25. Medicare
27. RA (Representative Assembly)
28. SLACK

30. JCAHO (Joint Commission on Accreditation of Health Organizations)
32. ICF (Intermediate Care Facility)
35. JOTS (*Journal of Occupational Therapy Students*)
36. Budget

Down

2. NA
4. Licensure
5. Salaries
6. PT (Physical Therapist)
7. AE (Above Elbow)
8. OTA (Occupational Therapy Assistant)
9. POTA (Pennsylvania Occupational Therapy Association)
12. SOAP (Subjective, Objective, Assessment, and Plan)

14. CAHEA (Committee on Allied Health Educational Accreditation)
15. Policy
18. Ad
19. AOTCB (American Occupational Therapy Certification Board)
20. CPR
22. AOTA (American Occupational Therapy Association)
24. DRG (Diagnostic Related Group)
26. Say AOTA
29. AMA (American Medical Association)
31. OT (Occupational Therapist)
33. AJOT (*American Journal of Occupational Therapy*)
34. WFOT (World Federation of Occupational Therapy)

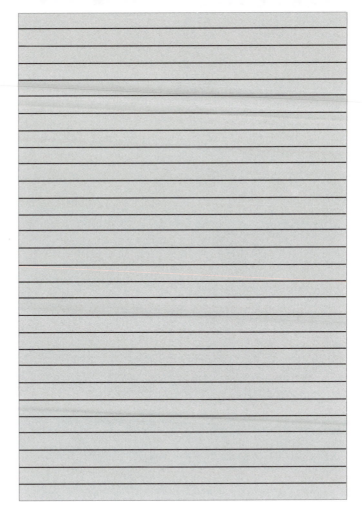

SECTION IV

Occupational Therapy Intervention

Part A

Pediatrics

Select the Most Appropriate Answer

1. A mentally retarded child can be trained to master a complex behavior by:
   A. Modeling
   B. Shaping
   C. Chaining
   D. Exploring

2. Circle the factor that should *not* be adhered to when engaging mentally retarded children in a low organizational game:
   A. Verbal instructions should be accompanied by demonstration
   B. Physical activities should be coordinated with music
   C. Instructions should be detailed and long
   D. Play periods should be frequent but short

3. The infant severely impaired by cerebral palsy requires assistance in experiencing his body and his environment; which of the following devices provides proper positioning?
   A. A wedge
   B. A prone board
   C. A corner chair
   D. All the above

4. A 13-year-old girl with rheumatoid arthritis since age 2 is referred to the occupational therapy (OT) department for joint protection techniques. She has moderate ulnar deviation of the fingers and wrists. Which activity is most contraindicated?
   A. Propelling her motorized wheelchair
   B. Crocheting
   C. Typing on an electric typewriter
   D. Squeezing a foam ball 10 times twice daily

5. The main responsibility of a certified occupational therapy assistant (COTA) in a mental retardation setting is:

    A. The performance of regular evaluations

    B. The construction and supervision of the use of orthoses

    C. The supervision of OT assistant students during Fieldwork II

    D. Attendance at department head meetings

6. Within OT intervention, lap feeding is used when:

    A. A child has poor head and trunk control

    B. A child does not want to sit on a chair

    C. A child wants to be closer to the therapist

    D. It is easier for the therapist

7. A child on a balance beam is being treated for one of the following problems:

    A. Hyperactivity

    B. Directionality

    C. Figure ground discrimination

    D. Astereognosis

The next three questions are based on the following information:

Tom is an 8-year-old boy who has been referred to OT because of an inability to read and write properly at his age group's expected level. A registered occupational therapist's (OTR's) evaluation identified very poor spatial relationships and motor planning abilities.

8. The initial treatment plan will emphasize:

    A. Spatial relationships

    B. Motor planning

    C. Handwriting skills

    D. Reading exercises

9. The appropriate testing procedure to evaluate the effects of treatment is one of the following:

    A. The Denver Developmental Screening test

    B. The manual muscle test

    C. The Sensory Integration Praxis test

    D. The Bruininks-Oseretsky Motor Developmental Scale

10. Tom is expected to have problems with:

    A.   Recalling facts
    B.   Tactile stimuli
    C.   Dressing skills
    D.   Riding a bus

11. A 6-year-old girl who isolates herself needs to improve socialization skills. Which of the following should be used first to meet her needs?

    A.   Games with small groups
    B.   Listening to the radio
    C.   Games with one other person
    D.   Games that she can play by herself

12. Which of the following activities would you use to increase the flexion of the shoulder to 90°, so that a child could put on his or her shirt independently?

    A.   Throwing clay on a potter wheel
    B.   Weaving on an inkle loom
    C.   Rug punching
    D.   Hanging string art on the wall

13. Tim, a 5-year-old below the elbow amputee who wears a prosthesis, has learned to use a pencil well. He was referred to OT to learn how to write his name. Initially, the therapist would expect the child to be able to:

    A.   Count to 200
    B.   Clean the prosthesis
    C.   Recognize numbers
    D.   Copy a square, circle, and triangle

14. Heavy joint compression is used in one of the following:

    A.   Brunnstrom approach
    B.   Vestibular stimulation
    C.   Proprioceptive facilitation technique
    D.   Bobath approach
    E.   Rood approach

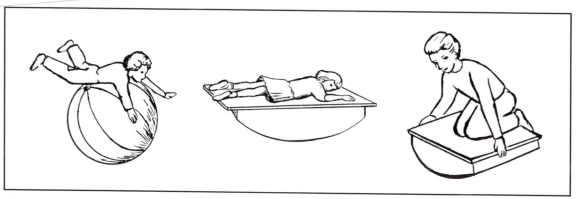

Figure 4-1.

15. The three children in these pictures have problems with (Figure 4-1):

    A. Motor planning
    B. Motor accuracy
    C. Equilibrium reactions
    D. Standing balance
    E. Body schema

16. The correct prehension pattern that a child uses when feeding himself or herself with a spoon is:

    A. Hook grasp
    B. Pincer grasp
    C. Three-point pinch
    D. Spherical grasp

17. One of the following is an example of symbolic play:

    A. Painting
    B. Silicone putty
    C. Dress up
    D. Hide and seek

18. A pediatric client with muscular dystrophy is included in a general program of exercise for one of the following reasons:

    A. To delay deterioration of cognitive abilities
    B. To prevent further weakness and incoordination
    C. To delay the development of deformities
    D. To prevent deformities

19. When assessing a child with feeding problems, the therapist should consider:
    A. Bite
    B. Mouth closure
    C. Chewing
    D. Swallowing
    E. All the above

20. The most realistic rehabilitative short-term goal for a 6-year-old girl with severe cerebral palsy who is wheelchair bound is to learn one of the following:
    A. To tie shoelaces
    B. Gait training
    C. Bed and wheelchair activities
    D. To make a ceramic project

21. When testing a 4-year-old boy with cerebral palsy for the development reflexive level, he displayed a positive reaction to the asymmetric tonic neck reflex. This means that when his head was turned to the side, the therapist observed:
    A. The flexion of the arm and leg on the skull side and/or an increase in flexor tone, and the extension of the arm and leg on the face side and/or an increase in extensor tone
    B. The flexion of both the upper and lower extremities
    C. The extension of the both the upper and lower extremities
    D. The flexion of the upper extremities and the extension of the lower extremities

22. A 6-year-old girl with cerebral palsy and hemiplegia is supine, and the therapist gives her an object to squeeze with the uninvolved hand. A mirroring and/or increase of muscle tone in the contralateral extremity occurs; the therapist observes the positive sign, within reflexive development, of one of the following:
    A. Tonic labyrinthine
    B. Withdrawal
    C. Symmetric tonic neck reflex
    D. Associated reactions

23. A 5-year-old child with cerebral palsy is supine, with his or her head in the midposition and arms and legs extended. The therapist, who is testing this patient for the level of reflexive development, rotates the patient's head to the side. The positive reaction of the neonatal neck and body righting reflex means that:
    A. The body rotates as a whole in the same direction
    B. The body rotates in the opposite direction
    C. The upper extremities flex and the lower extremities extend
    D. The body does not rotate

24. Substitution patterns of other groups of muscles to achieve the action of impaired muscles should be encouraged by the therapist when:
    A.   The affected muscles are graded poor minus
    B.   Minimal or no further recovery is expected
    C.   The impaired muscles are graded fair plus
    D.   Better results are expected immediately

25. A 6-year-old boy is having problems tying his shoelaces. Within normal development, this task is accomplished successfully when a child is:
    A.   5½ years of age
    B.   2½ years of age
    C.   4 years of age
    D.   2 years of age

26. A child was referred to OT to learn right-left discrimination. The therapist has to work toward the development of which of the following?
    A.   Laterality
    B.   Position in space
    C.   Directionality
    D.   Visual tracking

27. A child may have problems with laterality because:
    A.   He or she favors one side, completely ignoring the contralateral
    B.   The therapist tried to teach one-hand dominance
    C.   He or she mirrored every activity
    D.   A and C

28. Which of the following activities is more difficult for a child when using a pegboard in the training of form perception:
    A.   A vertical line on the left
    B.   A diagonal line
    C.   A vertical line on the board
    D.   A horizontal line in the right

29. When testing a child with perceptual motor impairment, the visual tracking area can be assessed by the therapist using one of the following:
    A.   An auditory counting test
    B.   A count the dot test
    C.   Picking out a specific number from a line of random numbers
    D.   B and C

30. A therapist is testing an 8-year-old child for kinesthetic ability by having the child:
    A. Write his or her name
    B. Identify familiar objects without visual cues
    C. Distinguish the difference between 1 lb and 3 lb sand bags
    D. Draw a square

31. Testing for hand dominance should be done when a child:
    A. Has problems with laterality
    B. Is under 3 years of age
    C. Routinely does not like to write or read
    D. Has problems with visual pursuit

32. When a child is jumping rope, the therapist expects him or her to receive what type(s) of sensory input?
    A. Visual
    B. Vestibular
    C. Proprioceptive
    D. All the above

33. When a therapist works with perceptually impaired children, he or she should:
    A. Expect that every child progresses at the same pace
    B. Expect marked improvement during the first 3 weeks of treatment
    C. Use a multisensory stimulation approach
    D. Stimulate not more than one sensory component at a time

34. Finger painting with shaving cream is a multisensory activity providing the following:
    A. Tactile stimuli
    B. Visual stimuli
    C. Auditory stimuli
    D. Olfactory stimuli
    E. A, B, and D

35. The therapist is evaluating a child for perceptual–motor impairment and identifies a problem with crossing the midline when:
    A. The child draws a very small circle when asked to draw a circle
    B. He or she draws a circle toward the dominant side
    C. The child draws a big circle
    D. He or she draws a circle toward the nondominant side

36. Turkish knotting on an upright frame is an appropriate activity:
    A. To enhance gross motor skills of the hands
    B. To increase socialization skills
    C. To obtain 120° of shoulder flexion
    D. To promote color discrimination

37. When evaluating sensory integrative and motor functions of a child, a therapist records data by:
    A. Gathering information from the parents
    B. Gathering information from other members of the professional team
    C. Observing motor behavior performance thoroughly
    D. Observing the child's interaction with other children
    E. All the above

38. A 6-year-old child was referred to OT, and upon thorough evaluation from the OTR, impairments in the following areas were identified:
    - Eye-hand coordination
    - Tactile and vestibular systems
    - Visual perception
    - Sensory processing
    - Academic difficulties referred by the teacher

    The therapist arrived at one of the following conclusions:
    A. Sensory integrative disorder
    B. Borderline mental retardation
    C. Mild form of childhood neurosis
    D. All the above

39. A 14-year-old boy suffered a spinal cord lesion at the T 5 to T 6 level. The most appropriate way to teach him how to put on his slacks is:
    A. Shifting weight from side to side when in a sitting position
    B. Sitting on the bed with his legs propped on a stool
    C. Rolling from one side to the other in bed
    D. Shifting weight from side to side when in a standing position

40. A therapist who uses play therapy when dealing with an abused child must recognize that:
    A. The therapist guides the therapy
    B. The setting of the play process guides the therapy sessions
    C. The child and the play guide the therapy
    D. The therapy is guided by the goals set by the professional team

41. For children with impaired neurological functions, which of the following is/are considered a common problem(s) when eating?

    A. Lip retraction
    B. Jaw thrust
    C. Tongue thrust
    D. All the above

42. Jaw control is a technique in which the care giver provides external stabilization to the child's jaw, controlling its opening and closing. This can be provided in two different approaches: front and side. Which of the following is the correct position when the therapist uses the front approach?

    A. The index finger on the front of the chin, the middle finger under the chin, the thumb on the side of the cheek
    B. The thumb in front of the chin, the middle finger under the chin, the index finger on the side of the cheek
    C. The index finger under the chin, the middle finger in front of the chin, the thumb on the side of the cheek
    D. The middle finger on the cheek, the thumb under the chin, and the index finger in front of the chin

43. When a child is referred to OT for handwriting problems, the therapist has to assess, among other things, "quality of movement." Which of the following is not under this category?

    A. Does the child maintain his or her head erect in the midline during writing?
    B. Are there motor planning impairments?
    C. Is writing movement stiff?
    D. Is there an automatic motion when writing?

44. A 7-year-old child has difficulty beginning and completing tasks in the classroom because of an auditory impairment in understanding and interpreting the spoken word. The OTR consultant should *not* recommend one of the following:

    A. Giving one direction at a time
    B. Decreasing auditory processing demands
    C. Increasing the amount of time to analyze the command
    D. A hearing aid

45. Billy is a boy with muscular dystrophy who is in a class for handicapped children. OT assessment shows poor dressing skills, poor hygienic care, dependency in self-feeding, good writing skills, weak but functional hand use, and difficulty with peer interaction. Which of the following is *not* an appropriate goal within OT intervention?

    A. Active participation in self-care activities
    B. Active participation in school curriculum appropriate to his intellectual abilities
    C. To encourage dependency in dressing skills to prevent further muscle weakness
    D. Active participation in play/leisure activities at school

46. Sherry is a 6-year-old girl who was referred to OT to maintain mental awareness and stimulate developmental play. One of the goals set was to enhance socialization and self-expression. In order to achieve this primary goal, using play therapy, which of the following is most desirable?

    A. Marbles
    B. Magazine picture collages
    C. Riding a tricycle
    D. Putting a simple puzzle together

47. Initially, the treatment of a patient who is tactile defensive is:

    A. Teaching safety measures
    B. Teaching substitution patterns
    C. Teaching compensatory measures
    D. Desensitization techniques

48. If a child has a perceptual problem in the kinesthetic and tactile areas, one of the modes of OT intervention is to:

    A. Touch the body parts to be moved
    B. Tell the patient about the movie seen on television
    C. Give short verbal directions to the patient
    D. Use visual aids in training procedures

49. During the evaluation of a child with hemiplegia, the occupational therapist asks the child to copy a circle and a square to assess one of the following:

    A. Nystagmus
    B. Motor skills of the upper extremity
    C. Perception
    D. Intellectual abilities

50. When a therapist asks a hemiplegic child to identify a familiar object in the involved hand without visual clues, he or she is assessing:

    A. Agraphia
    B. Proprioception
    C. Alexia
    D. Stereognosis

51. Considering motor development, which of the following statements is *not* true?

    A. The maturation of shoulder muscles precedes the maturation of hand muscles
    B. Normal development occurs from a lateral direction to a medial direction
    C. Rotation is the last movement to be developed
    D. Normal development occurs from ulnar to radial

52. A 14-year-old boy has neuropathy of the radial nerve with the extensor group graded fair. A therapist may begin:

    A. Antigravity exercises
    B. Antigravity plus maximal resistance exercises
    C. Exercises with gravity eliminated
    D. Antigravity plus moderate resistance exercises

53. Puppetry is a media used in pediatric psychiatric OT. Which of the following is more readily used to stimulate projection techniques?

    A. A rod puppet
    B. A glove puppet
    C. A shadow puppet
    D. A marionette

54. A child who is able to differentiate right from left but cannot identify body parts has an impairment with:

    A. Directionality
    B. Body scheme
    C. Motor planning
    D. Visual pursuit

55. A client bumps into objects/furniture when walking because of a deficit in judging distances. This child has an impairment in which of the following areas:

    A. Right-left discrimination
    B. Topographical orientation
    C. Spatial relations
    D. Position in space

56. The COTA is performing the motor analysis of an activity to be given to a child. Which of the following is the best approach?

    A. Biomechanical
    B. Neurodevelopmental
    C. Sensory
    D. A and B

57. A COTA is analyzing a therapeutic activity seeking for the sensory, perceptual, and physical components. This type of analysis is:

    A. Biomechanical
    B. Sensory integrative
    C. Ontogenetic
    D. Phylogenetic

58. A COTA working in a pediatric setting is performing self-care activities with an 8-year-old child who has limited range of motion. The treatment plan includes:

    A. Changing body mechanics
    B. Increasing the child's reach
    C. Providing stability
    D. Increasing sensory awareness

59. A therapist is working with a 6-month-old infant who shows neck asymmetry. Which group of muscles needs to be primarily developed?

    A. Flexors
    B. Hyperextensors
    C. Rotators
    D. Abductors

60. A 3-year-old child needs to increase arm strength. The COTA is giving a finger-painting activity placing the working surface:

    A. At elbow height
    B. At shoulder height
    C. Inclined upwards
    D. Inclined downwards

61. Position and motion sense can be tested by one of the following methods:
    A. The recognition of common objects by sense of touch alone
    B. The identification of position change of body parts, without visual cues when performed by someone other than the patient
    C. The recognition of numbers, letters, and forms written on the skin with occluded vision
    D. The recognition of cold and hot objects without the use of the vision sense

62. Among the following activities, which one facilitates extension of the vertebral column?
    A. Crawling on a carpeted floor
    B. Riding a scooter board in a prone position
    C. Walking through a maze
    D. Riding a seesaw

63. A child who had a recent head injury has sequencing problems. Which approach will be more appropriate within OT intervention?
    A. Isolate each of the various steps of the activity
    B. Identify different options for the completion of the activity
    C. Provide verbal directions
    D. Demonstrate the performance of the activity in its entirety

64. When a therapist is constructing a hand splint for a child with a burn, he or she should:
    A. Meet the exact custom needs of the child
    B. Keep the design simple
    C. Keep the wrist between neutral and 30° of dorsiflexion
    D. Avoid any inappropriate pressure
    E. All the above

65. Which of the following is more appropriate for a 2-year-old child?
    A. Colorful, large, three-dimensional toys
    B. A scooter board
    C. Toys with no removable parts
    D. Toys requiring a great deal of manual dexterity

66. Toys can be used to elicit specific patterns/movements. Select the toy that mostly encourages the prone extension pattern:
    A. A rolling pin
    B. A scooter board
    C. Puppets
    D. A balloon blower

67. Usually the infant younger than 6 months enjoys playing with:

    A.   Small blocks
    B.   Strings of snap beads
    C.   Rattles of various shapes and colors
    D.   Water

68. Which of the following is most likely to meet the needs of a 2-year-old child?

    A.   A toy bus
    B.   Blocks
    C.   A scooter board
    D.   A four-piece puzzle

69. A 15-year-old girl with mild to moderate depression was given a ball of clay in the OT clinic. Thirty minutes later a sculpture of *The Thinker* sitting on the top of a rock emerged. Which of the following was demonstrated?

    A.   Projective technique
    B.   Cooperative play technique
    C.   Parallel play technique
    D.   None of the above

70. As a treatment modality, music provides experiences within a structure that stimulate sensory behavior by:

    A.   Demanding reality-oriented behavior
    B.   Demanding immediate and objectified behavior
    C.   Allowing the ordering of behavior according to the physical response level
    D.   Demanding increased sensory image and discrimination

71. When treating children with mental retardation, the therapist must establish:

    A.   Goals with average expectations
    B.   Goals that are realistic given the level of retardation
    C.   Goals that require a moderate level of frustration
    D.   Goals that nullify self-esteem

72. Which of the following is handled more easily by a child with hemiplegia?

    A.   Front-opening garments
    B.   Back-opening garments
    C.   Side-opening garments
    D.   A combination of the three

Part B

Physical Dysfunction

Select the Most Appropriate Answer

1. According to some experts, work hardening is an adjustment activity that focuses on the reacquisition of skills and work habits to ensure job success. These elements include:

   A. Punctuality
   B. Appropriate acceptance of supervision
   C. Interpersonal relationships
   D. The ability to ask for assistance when necessary
   E. B, C, and D
   F. All the above

2. Which of the following instruments is most useful in selecting an appropriate game or hobby for a 72-year-old patient in a nursing home?

   A. A test on perceptual abilities
   B. An interest questionnaire
   C. A range of motion (ROM) test
   D. A manual muscle test

3. A 42-year-old housewife with paraplegia is referred to occupational therapy (OT) for home evaluation. The therapist recommends:

   A. A side by side refrigerator
   B. The counters and the stove top should be at wheelchair level
   C. The kitchen should be arranged following this sequence: refrigerator, sink, stove
   D. All the above

4. A patient with a Colles' fracture should avoid:

   A. Bilateral activities
   B. Activities that involve shoulder motion
   C. Sustained positions of the hand
   D. Stress management activities

5. Which of the following activities is most appropriate for a rheumatoid arthritic client?

A. A needlepoint pillow
B. A tile trivet
C. Modelling clay
D. Copper tooling

6. Copper tooling is an activity contraindicated for patients with:

A. Respiratory dysfunctions
B. Psychosomatic dysfunctions
C. Borderline mental retardation
D. All the above

7. A man with a recent head injury has a problem with sequencing. The best treatment method is to:

A. Verbally explain the procedure several times
B. Give the patient written instructions to follow
C. Demonstrate procedures to the patient slowly
D. Isolate the individual steps of the activity

8. The OT motto, work hardening, means an individual will reenter the work force at his or her highest possible level of functioning that includes:

A. The achievement of optimal physical reconditioning
B. The identification of problems and possible solutions
C. The facilitation of maximal psychosocial and cognitive skills
D. All the above
E. A and B only

9. When teaching a patient with hemiplegia to propel his or her own wheelchair:

A. Remove the footrest from the uninvolved side and begin with the patient using both unaffected extremities
B. The client must be able to use both upper extremities
C. Defer training until the appropriate one-arm-drive wheelchair is available
D. The client is taught to push backwards with the involved leg and pull forward with the unaffected leg

10. The most important component of the rehabilitation program for the right above elbow amputee is learning:

    A. To incorporate the new limb substitute within his or her body's schema
    B. To take care of the prosthesis
    C. To use feeding utensils
    D. To learn how to lock and unlock the elbow joint

11. The first step in teaching a left below elbow amputee to don a front-opening shirt is one of the following:

    A. Put the garment on the amputated side first
    B. Pull the garment overhead
    C. Put the garment on the sound arm first
    D. Put the garment on both arms simultaneously

12. The homemaker with hemiplegia may be advised by the occupational therapist to:

    A. Use one-handed pots and pans
    B. Use heavier cookware to compensate for impaired sensation
    C. Examine oneself for burns because of diminished sensation of the involved upper extremity
    D. A and C

13. A patient with rheumatoid arthritis has significant ulnar drift at the metacarpophalangeal joints (MCPJs). One of the following OT interventions can be used:

    A. A cock-up hand splint
    B. Device forcing fingers toward radial deviation
    C. A resting pan hand splint
    D. None the above

14. When teaching a man who has had a cerebrovascular accident (CVA) to propel his wheelchair, the therapist must tell him to use:

    A. The uninvolved leg and involved arm
    B. The involved leg and involved arm
    C. The uninvolved leg and uninvolved arm
    D. The involved leg and uninvolved arm

15. When a 54-year-old patient with hemiparesia is putting on a front-opening shirt, he should:

    A. Put the involved arm into the sleeve first
    B. Put the uninvolved arm into the sleeve first
    C. Put both arms into the sleeves simultaneously
    D. Pull the garment over his head

16. When a 54-year-old patient with hemiparesia is removing a front-opening shirt, he should:
    A. Remove the involved arm first
    B. Remove the uninvolved arm first
    C. Remove the normal arm last
    D. Ask for assistance

17. In a work hardening setting, the therapist teaches a client the proper method to carry a heavy load. Good advice is to:
    A. Hold the load as close to the body as possible
    B. Avoid transporting the load on a wheelchair
    C. Keep the back arched during the transportation of the load
    D. Rotate at the trunk rather than turning the whole body

18. When the certified occupational therapy assistant (COTA) plans activities for the rheumatoid arthritic patient, he or she must focus on:
    A. Maintaining the range of wrist extension and forearm supination
    B. Encouraging activities involving a strong grasp as well as ulnar deviation
    C. Teaching the patient to grasp objects diagonally across the palm
    D. Emphasizing finger dexterity, such as knitting

19. A patient with hemiplegia is learning transfer techniques. When transferring from the wheel-chair to the bathtub, he or she should:
    A. Use a straight-back chair inside the bathtub
    B. Bear weight only on the affected side
    C. Bear weight only on the unaffected side
    D. Place the wheelchair facing the tub directly

20. The COTA's initial action toward a woman with a recent amputation who appears to be moderately depressed should be to:
    A. Send the patient back to her room
    B. Report the situation to the supervisor immediately
    C. Introduce the patient to a simple activity of the patient's liking
    D. Review the patient's chart for updated information before proceeding

21. A 30-year-old patient with hemiplegia is referred to OT to increase homemaking skills. Which of the following equipment would be the most useful?
    A. Bowl stabilizer
    B. Pots with bilateral handles
    C. Long-handled utensils
    D. Built-up handled utensils

22. The most important components that the COTA should report to the supervisor after observing the work performance of a patient with a physical dysfunction are:
    A. Work habits, manual dexterity, and endurance
    B. Creativity, enthusiasm, and enjoyment of the job
    C. Sociability, leadership skills, and interest in career
    D. Strength, educational level, grooming habits, and coordination

23. A client will benefit the most from a work-simplification program in homemaking if these tasks become automatic. The best method to do this is to:
    A. Allow family members to help the client in the performance of activities
    B. Give appropriate adaptive equipment to increase the patient's independence
    C. Identify the techniques and their steps, and practice each activity repeatedly
    D. Involve family members in the performance of activities under the therapist's supervision

24. Avocational interests with spinal cord injury patients are to be explored as part of the rehabilitation process to:
    A. Give patients leisure opportunities
    B. Give patients something to do upon discharge from the hospital
    C. Take the patient's mind off his or her own problems
    D. Alleviate the family's concerns after discharge

25. A man who had a stroke without medical complications should be out of bed within 24 to 48 hours after a cerebral thrombosis. Therefore, he should:
    A. Not be required to begin any type of activity
    B. Be lifted onto a wheelchair until more time has passed by
    C. Immediately be encouraged to use the involved side for feeding, toileting, transferring, etc.
    D. Be left alone until he is "ready" to initiate any activities of daily living (ADL)

26. A woman with a lower extremity prosthesis went shopping. What can she use in the place of her walker/cane/crutch?
    A. A stand
    B. Shelves
    C. A shopping cart
    D. Assistance from another person

27. When a therapist is treating a patient with a coronary condition, he or she should watch for:
    A. Signs of euphoria
    B. Accommodation
    C. Signs of fatigue
    D. Vertigo

28. When training a man with a lower extremity prosthesis how to use the bus, which is usually *not* a responsibility of the OT department?
    A. Deciding where to put ambulatory equipment while giving the fare to the driver
    B. Practicing going up and down the steps
    C. Determining which side of the bus is easier to sit on
    D. Getting on the bus

29. The most suitable type of refrigerator for the wheelchair bound homemaker is:
    A. Freezer compartment on the top
    B. Side by side
    C. Freezer compartment on the bottom
    D. Counter top

30. Considering work-simplification techniques, which of the following activities is *not* recommended for coronary patients?
    A. Use one hand rather than two
    B. Sit rather than stand while working
    C. Use a long-handled dusting pan
    D. Eliminate unnecessary tasks
    E. Finish all activities in one area before moving to another

31. Within work-simplification techniques, which of the following is *not* advisable for cardiac patients?
    A. Lift all pans and other objects as opposed to sliding them
    B. Store all utensils at the point of first use
    C. Use suction cups to hold bowls while mixing foods
    D. Use a bathtub seat
    E. Use a wheeled cart to transport laundry and dirty dishes

32. Mr. G, a 45-year-old man with left hemiplegia, is in treatment in the OT Clinic. The COTA observes the patient experiencing perspiration and heavy breathing. The therapist should:

    A. Call a nurse immediately
    B. Allow the patient to rest briefly and observe the signs
    C. Continue with activity to increase endurance
    D. Begin emergency procedures

33. A patient comes to the OT clinic with a wrist and thumb drop. This deformity occurs in which peripheral nerve injury?

    A. Brachial plexus
    B. Axillary
    C. Radial
    D. Median

34. A 66-year-old man with right hemiplegia is referred to OT for ADL evaluation and training. What is the first step the therapist should take?

    A. Give him a dressing aid
    B. Have him take off his shirt only
    C. Engage in meaningful conversation
    D. Let him attempt dressing skills while the therapist observes

35. When the COTA explains OT intervention to the client and the client's family, the COTA should *not:*

    A. Explain why the services are recommended for the client
    B. Explain what the goals of the treatment process are
    C. Explain what the treatment process will be and the reason why
    D. Explain in detail one's own background, school attended, marital status, age, etc.

36. A patient with a spinal cord injury should be initiated in ADL training:

    A. While the patient is still in bed
    B. After the patient has had a few treatments in physical therapy
    C. After the patient attends 2 to 3 sessions in the OT clinic
    D. After the patient starts specific graded activities

37. An individual diagnosed as a C4 quadriplegic has little muscle power left. In order for him or her to achieve the status of functioning at a productive level, one of the following is necessary:

   A.   Assistive exercise
   B.   Increased ROM
   C.   Increased strength
   D.   External power

38. Patients with spinal cord injuries, after being evaluated in the homemaking area, need to be taught:

   A.   Labor-saving methods
   B.   Energy-conservation techniques
   C.   Work-simplification techniques
   D.   All the above

39. An arm sling may be used to support the flaccid extremity to prevent shoulder subluxation. Which of the following forces is a concern for the therapist when the patient ambulates wearing the sling?

   A.   The strength of the elbow muscles
   B.   The strength of the forearm muscles and the elbow muscles
   C.   Gravity
   D.   Spasticity

40. When transferring a paraplegic patient from wheelchair to bed, the first step after positioning is to:

   A.   Lift foot rests
   B.   Place feet on the floor 6 inches apart
   C.   Lock the wheels of the wheelchair
   D.   Scoot forward in the wheelchair

41. When a therapist performs passive ROM to the right upper extremity of a patient with a left CVA, the main goal(s) is/are:

   A.   Increase stiffness of the joints
   B.   Decrease pain
   C.   Decrease stiffness and increase ROM
   D.   None the above

42. A woman diagnosed as having a CVA lacks active motion in her affected upper extremity, although she shows moderate to maximal improvement in sitting balance. When the COTA reports this to the supervisor, he or she should indicate that patient may be able to:

    A.   Make her own bed
    B.   Begin gait training
    C.   Partially sponge bathe herself without assistance
    D.   Use the bathroom facilities independently

43. An active 47-year-old man who had a myocardial infarction 3 weeks ago has been referred to OT. When performing the initial evaluation of self-care skills, it is very important to:

    A.   Help the client in any tasks he cannot do independently
    B.   Ask him what he would like to do independently
    C.   Observe for any possible physical discomfort
    D.   Inquire about the physical layout of the rooms in his home

44. A 60-year-old confused woman has a right hemiplegia, and the COTA is teaching her how to dress independently. The first step should be:

    A.   Demonstrate the techniques
    B.   Verbally explain the different steps of dressing
    C.   Break down the activity into smaller steps
    D.   Have another patient simultaneously perform dressing techniques

45. When the therapist assesses the patient's employability potential, the most important factor to consider is:

    A.   Physical strength
    B.   Coordination
    C.   Cognitive capabilities
    D.   Work habits

46. An 18-year-old man has a complete transection of the spinal cord at the T5, T6 level. Prior to working on transfer techniques, which of the following should be strengthened?

    A.   The upper portion of the trapezius
    B.   The biceps
    C.   The latissimus dorsi
    D.   The serratus anterior

47. The best method for a 17-year-old boy with a spinal cord injury at the T6 level to put on his trousers is to:
    A. Sit on a regular chair with his legs propped on a stool
    B. Sit over the side of a bed with his legs resting on a foot stool
    C. Roll in bed from side to side
    D. Shift his weight from side to side when sitting in a wheelchair

48. When using braid weaving with a woman with hemiplegia whose involved right shoulder flexion is graded fair, the involved upper extremity must be:
    A. Resting on the lap
    B. Resting on a triangle sling
    C. Suspended on a deltoid aid (overhead arm sling)
    D. Strapped to the beater

49. Which of the following is the most important factor to consider when training a 35-year-old homemaker with hemiplegia?
    A. An adaptive kitchen
    B. Time and energy conservation techniques
    C. A change of hand dominance
    D. Adaptive equipment

50. When teaching ADL to a patient with hemiplegia, the most important factor for successful training is:
    A. Good rapport between the patient and the therapist
    B. The patient's motivation to become independent
    C. The patient's good communication skills
    D. The therapist clearly presents tasks to the patient

51. A 65-year-old homemaker with Parkinson's disease should be encouraged to:
    A. Wear gloves to reduce intention tremor
    B. Use heavy pots and pans in the kitchen to decrease tremors
    C. Stop all activities outside the house
    D. Delete most homemaking activities

52. A woman with a peripheral neuropathy referred to OT was initially evaluated and found to be unable to extend her thumb. She had a sensory impairment on the dorsal surface of the thumb, and the second and third fingers on the proximal phalanx. These are signs of a peripheral nerve injury of the:

    A. Ulnar nerve
    B. Musculocutaneous nerve
    C. Radial nerve
    D. Median nerve

53. A bilateral above the knee amputee needs to transfer to the toilet seat. The best method to train him or her is one of the following:

    A. Using a wheelchair with an opening back rest, approach the back of the wheelchair to the front of the toilet seat, lock the wheelchair, and slide back using push-ups
    B. Place the wheelchair parallel to the toilet (side approach), lock the wheelchair, and slide sideways using push-ups
    C. Place the wheelchair at a 90° angle with the toilet, lock the wheelchair, use push-ups, and pivot toward the toilet
    D. The wheelchair faces the toilet seat, the patient transfers to the toilet, then turns around on the seat to face forward

54. The best method to mobilize stiff joints in the hand is:

    A. Forceful exercises performed by a therapist
    B. Active exercises several times a day
    C. Daily heat treatments
    D. Self-forceful exercises to tolerance

55. When evaluating a Parkinsonian patient, a therapist may observe which of the following:

    A. Rigidity
    B. Loss of sensation
    C. Bradykinesia
    D. A and C

56. When the registered occupational therapist evaluates a patient with multiple sclerosis, he or she may find:

    A. Tremors
    B. Speech problems
    C. Muscle weakness
    D. All the above

57. A person with a spinal cord injury at the T1 level would benefit from the use of:
    A. A standard wheelchair
    B. Built-up handles
    C. A mobile arm support
    D. A deltoid aid

58. A quadriplegic man "blacked out" while in the OT department. Because he had just begun to sit in a wheelchair, the therapist should:
    A. Tilt the patient back, and elevate his legs
    B. Call a doctor or nurse
    C. Give him a drink of water
    D. Take the patient back to his room

59. A right CVA patient has the wrist extensors on the involved hand graded trace. The therapist's primary consideration should be to:
    A. Encourage prehension with the wrist in flexion
    B. Wear a splint with the wrist continually in 20° dorsiflexion
    C. Encourage grasp with the wrist in midposition
    D. Not permit the wrist to be positioned in extreme flexion

60. Within stroke rehabilitation, a therapist may expect the patients to:
    A. Have permanent pain in the involved hand
    B. Have complete recovery of hand function
    C. Accept the idea of not being able to use either hand
    D. Use the affected hand as a helper

61. A woman who received her upper extremity prosthesis for the first time should leave it in the OT clinic after her first session until she:
    A. Can don and remove the prosthesis independently
    B. Has no skin irritation
    C. Has completed use training
    D. Has the prosthesis checked for fit and comfort

62. Within OT intervention, the initial assessment of self-maintenance of a patient includes the:
    A. Patient's present income and how it is managed
    B. Ability to perform activities taught in the OT clinic
    C. Patient's present hospital insurance coverage
    D. Necessary activities to maintain life support needs

63. When dealing with the geriatric population (people over 65) during activity planning, the therapist has to make the patient aware of one of the following:

    A.   Correct activities generate sufficient energy to minimize tiring
    B.   Old patterns of life cannot be used continually
    C.   New patterns of life need to be initiated
    D.   Working hard in OT will overcome most handicaps

64. When transferring a patient with quadriplegia, "good" neck musculature, "poor" shoulder muscles, and "zero" elbow muscles, the therapist must teach the:

    A.   Pivot transfer
    B.   Hydraulic lift transfer
    C.   Bobath method transfer
    D.   Sliding board transfer

65. A patient with quadriplegia with fair shoulder muscles and fair elbow flexion should be transferred by using one of the following techniques:

    A.   Pivot transfer
    B.   Sliding board transfer
    C.   Bobath method transfer
    D.   Lift transfer

66. When implementing a cardiac rehabilitation program, the therapist should educate the:

    A.   Certified Nursing Assistant who works with the patient
    B.   Occupational therapy assistant student
    C.   Patient
    D.   Patient and family

67. During an evaluation of a patient with hemiplegia, the therapist gives the client single geometric figures to copy (e.g., square, circle). The therapist is mainly assessing:

    A.   Topographic orientation
    B.   Perception
    C.   Cognition
    D.   Memory

68. Following a total hip replacement, a patient must use:

    A.   An abduction wedge between the legs
    B.   A reclining wheelchair for hip flexion precautions
    C.   A raised commode seat to meet bathroom needs
    D.   All the above

69. When planning a treatment program for a patient with low back pain, the therapist will include:

    A. Teaching appropriate body mechanics
    B. Patient education
    C. Good standing and sitting postures
    D. All the above

70. In OT intervention, activity restriction and work-simplification techniques are termed:

    A. Positioning
    B. Joint protection
    C. Energy conservation
    D. Work hardening

71. Considering OT intervention, the minimization of stress for prevention of deformities is called:

    A. Positioning
    B. Joint protection
    C. Energy conservation
    D. Splinting

72. For a patient who has a dysfunction as a result of immaturity of the central nervous system, and some improvement is expected, which of the following treatment approaches should be selected?

    A. Rehabilitative
    B. Neurodevelopmental
    C. Neurobiological
    D. Psychological

73. Upon reevaluation of a radial nerve injury, the therapist graded the extensors *fair*. The patient is ready to begin:

    A. Antigravity exercises
    B. Exercises with the help of gravity
    C. Powder board exercise, with gravity eliminated as much as possible
    D. Exercises against gravity, plus minimal resistance

74. In manual muscle testing, the expression "maximal resistance" means:
    A. The maximum amount of time the patient is able to tolerate maximal resistance from the therapist
    B. The maximal effort that the patient is capable of performing in a given movement
    C. The maximal resistance the patient is able to sustain and overcome successfully
    D. The maximal resistance the therapist is able to apply to the patient

75. Considering the patient with hemiplegia, rotation of the trunk inhibits:
    A. Flaccidity of the involved side
    B. Normal muscle tone bilaterally
    C. Spasticity on the involved side
    D. Leaning the trunk toward the stronger side

76. During assessment, a therapist measures the flexion of the MCPJ of the last four fingers of the right hand from 0° to 45°. This measurement means that there is:
    A. No limitation in flexion of the fingers
    B. Limitation of the fingers at the MCPJs is present
    C. Limitation in finger extension at the MCPJ
    D. Limitation in the MCPJ abduction at the MCPJ

77. When a patient has the right triceps graded F-(3-), a short term goal will be to:
    A. Improve strength to fair (3)
    B. Improve strength to F+(3+)
    C. Improve strength to G-(4-)
    D. Improve strength to good +(4+)

78. A stroke patient is about to be discharged from the hospital. Considering architectural barriers, a home evaluation is in order after the identification of possible problems by the:
    A. Doctor
    B. Occupational therapist
    C. Patient's family
    D. Therapist and patient

79. The practice of good body mechanics, energy conservation techniques, weight reduction instructions, and relaxation techniques are most likely used in which of the following programs:

    A. Vocational training
    B. Work hardening
    C. Prevocational and training
    D. Stress management

80. The evaluation of a CVA patient should begin with which of the following areas:

    A. Self-care
    B. ROM
    C. Perceptual motor
    D. Muscle strength and coordination

81. When performing a sensory evaluation of a patient with hemiplegia, the therapist will first test:

    A. The involved side
    B. The uninvolved side
    C. Either way
    D. Both simultaneously
    E. Neither

82. Which of the following should *not* be performed by a rheumatoid arthritic patient?

    A. Minimal to moderate resistive activities
    B. Activities that maintain a specific position for a prolonged period of time
    C. Gentle activities with periods of rest
    D. Activities within the limits of pain

83. A patient who suffered severe burns must be splinted to prevent deformities and contractures of the burned area(s) as soon as:

    A. The patient has been admitted to the hospital
    B. The edema stage is in progress
    C. The pain in the involved area decreases
    D. The grafting in the burned area is well-healed

84. The sequence of the rehabilitation process for an amputee is as follows:

    A. Amputation—preprosthetic treatment (when necessary)—preprosthetic evaluation—prescription

    B. Amputation—training—initial checkout—prosthetic evaluation—prescription—fabrication of prosthesis—prosthetic training—final checkout

    C. Amputation—preprosthetic evaluation—preprosthetic treatment (when necessary)—prescription—fabrication—initial checkout—training—final checkout

    D. Amputation—prescription—preprosthetic treatment—preprosthetic evaluation—prescription—fabrication—training—initial checkout—final checkout

85. When a patient with an above the elbow amputation comes to the OT clinic, the first body motions to be taught are:

    A. Open/close terminal device (TD)

    B. Lock/unlock elbow unit

    C. Elbow flexion/extension forearm lift and open/close TD

    D. Supination/pronation

86. When an above the elbow amputee performs shoulder flexion on the amputated side with the elbow locked, which of the following takes place?

    A. Supination of the TD

    B. Pronation of the TD

    C. Unlocking of the elbow

    D. Opening of the TD

87. It is essential that burned patients perform active movements everyday, several times a day, to prevent deformities. These exercises must begin:

    A. The first day of the acute phase

    B. When skin grafting is healed

    C. When it is no longer painful

    D. The day of admission

88. The initial prosthetic checkout on a client should be accomplished:

    A. Between controls training and use training

    B. After the patient begins use training

    C. Before the patient begins use training

    D. On the second day of controls training

89. Some patients seen at bedside are in traction. Traction is one of the following:

    A. A nonconservative treatment in low back pain (LBP)
    B. A conservative treatment in LBP
    C. A contraindicated treatment in LBP
    D. Definitive treatment specific for LBP

90. One of the following activities is contraindicated for muscle strengthening:

    A. Knitting
    B. Gardening
    C. Woodworking
    D. Leather tooling

91. Side neglect can be illustrated by a patient with hemiplegia when he or she is asked to draw:

    A. A clock
    B. Geometric figures
    C. A person's body
    D. Animals

92. When the COTA evaluates a patient for ADL, the primary objective is to:

    A. Gather, analyze, and interpret pertinent information
    B. Determine the patient's interests
    C. Establish a good rapport with the patient
    D. Talk with other members of the professional team

93. A COTA constructed a cock-up splint and fitted it to the patient's hand. The splint was worn for 30 minutes, and the therapist spotted a red area, which was apparent for 45 minutes. What should the COTA do?

    A. Reapply the splint after the 45 minutes
    B. Pad the area on the splint that produced the redness
    C. Construct a new splint
    D. Reevaluate the splint to ensure less pressure in the area that produced redness

94. The COTA was performing ROM at bedside and discovered a broken skin area at the elbow. He or she should:

    A. Inform the patient's certified nursing assistant
    B. Report the situation to the supervisor
    C. Mention it to the patient
    D. Give the patient directions in skin self-care

95. For patients with aphasia resulting from a CVA, injury was most likely:
    A. On the dominant side of the brain
    B. On the nondominant side of the brain
    C. On the dominant side of the body
    D. Always in the left hemisphere

96. When working with patients with hemiplegia, the areas of the body that will have the least functional return are the:
    A. Knee and ankle
    B. Elbow and foot
    C. Hand and fingers
    D. Shoulder and elbows

97. Mobile arm supports are sophisticated pieces of equipment used in OT clinics with which of the following?
    A. Patients with peripheral nerve injuries
    B. Patients with Parkinson's disease
    C. Patients with paraplegia
    D. Patients with quadriplegia and older patients with poliomyelitis

98. The COTA reads in the patient's chart the goniometric measurement of elbow flexion is 20° to 135°. This means:
    A. There is no limitation in the ROM of the elbow joint
    B. There is limitation in extension of the elbow joint
    C. There is limitation in flexion
    D. There is limitation in both flexion and extension of the elbow joint

99. When treating a patient with a chronic condition, for which no improvement is expected, what approaches should be used?
    A. Neurodevelopmental
    B. Psychosocial
    C. Rehabilitative
    D. Biomechanical

100. Which of the following is the best activity to encourage trunk stability in the brain damaged adult?
    A. Lying supine and doing crafts
    B. Lying on the side and doing crafts
    C. Sitting and performing table activities
    D. Bilateral sawing and sanding

101. During OT intervention, the COTA noticed that the active ROM of the elbow was less than the passive ROM. This is a sign of:

    A. Limitation of ROM
    B. Muscle weakness
    C. Contracture
    D. Muscle incoordination

102. A patient with "claw hand" was referred to the OT clinic. The experienced clinician knows that this deformity is commonly seen in one of the following peripheral nerve injuries:

    A. Median nerve
    B. Radial nerve
    C. Ulnar nerve
    D. Musculocutaneous nerve
    E. Axillary nerve

103. When splinting an injured hand, the therapist in the majority of the cases must keep the wrist in functional position:

    A. Approximately 15° in flexion
    B. Approximately 30° in dorsiflexion
    C. Approximately 20° in flexion
    D. Approximately 10° in dorsiflexion

104. When the therapist constructs a cock-up hand splint, the palmar piece should not go beyond the:

    A. Proximal interphalangeal joints
    B. MCPJs
    C. Distal palmar crease
    D. Proximal palmar crease

105. A patient diagnosed as a right CVA with a resultant left hemiparesis was assigned to a COTA working in a general hospital setting. While examining the client's chart, the COTA reads that the left upper extremity has *fair* to *good* muscle power. This information indicates:

    A. Poor ROM measurement
    B. Grades of manual muscle testing
    C. Poor prognosis for recovery
    D. No active movement is present

The next 20 questions (106 to 125) concern physical agent modalities, which since 1992 have been formally administered within segments of the OT profession.

106. The following effects are most likely to result from the use of therapeutic heat as a physical agent modality (PAM), with *one exception*:
    A. Prevention of soft tissue contractures
    B. Decrease in joint stiffness
    C. Increase in local circulation
    D. Alleviation of painful stimuli

107. This PAM is *least* likely to be useful in treating hand conditions:
    A. Paraffin
    B. Ultraviolet light
    C. Whirlpool
    D. Fluidotherapy

108. This PAM, because of its specific heat, is used as a treatment agent in the temperature range of 128° to 132° F (53° to 55.5° C):
    A. Hot packs
    B. Whirlpool bath
    C. Fluidotherapy cabinet
    D. Paraffin dip

109. Which of the following is *not* an advantage in using the whirlpool bath as the physical modality of choice?
    A. Wound cleansing is possible, because of the effect of moving water
    B. Circumferential treatment of the immersed body part occurs
    C. The patient is able to move or exercise a body part, if desired, during treatment
    D. Higher tissue temperatures can be maintained than with the use of other modalities

110. When a paralyzed muscle is being treated with little likelihood of any functional return, the type of electrical stimulation most often considered is:
    A. Faradic current
    B. Sinusoidal, (alternating) current
    C. Low voltage galvanic (direct) current
    D. High voltage galvanic current

111. When applying ultrasound via direct contact, using the continuous mode, which factor regarding technique is *incorrect*?

    A. A coupling agent is always used
    B. Patient comfort is unreliable, as to dosage intensity of ultrasound
    C. The sound head is kept in motion
    D. The sound head motions partially overlap tissue, as it is moved along during treatment

112. Which statement about ultrasound diathermy, or ultrasound, is *not* correct?

    A. Ultrasound may be used both continuously and pulsed (intermittently)
    B. Ultrasound may be administered under water
    C. Ultrasound is believed to have both thermal and nonthermal effects
    D. Ultrasonic diathermy and short wave diathermy are essentially similar

113. Which statement regarding the use of hot packs as a PAM is *not* correct?

    A. Hot packs provide conductive heating of tissues
    B. With normal circulation and sensation, the danger of overheating is minimal
    C. The hot pack is positioned away from direct skin contact by the use of multiple layers of toweling
    D. Hot packs commonly in use contain a water-absorbing silica gel

114. A properly written prescription, ordering physical agent modalities, should *not* include the following information:

    A. The patient's name and age
    B. The patient's marital status
    C. Area(s) to be treated
    D. Any special instructions

115. With the standard manual muscle test (MMT), an individual muscle was given a grade of trace. This means:

    A. The ROM is complete, against gravity
    B. There is no detectable evidence of muscle contraction
    C. There is evidence of muscle contraction, but no joint motion is detected
    D. The ROM is complete, with one likely exception.

116. Hydrocollator packs may be prescribed for the treatment of all of the following conditions, with one likely exception:

    A. Peripheral vascular disease
    B. Bursitis
    C. Osteo/rheumatoid arthritis
    D. Relief of muscle spasm

117. One of the following conditions is a definite contraindication for the use of paraffin:

    A.   Rheumatoid/osteoarthritis

    B.   Arteriosclerosis

    C.   Diabetes mellitus

    D.   Open wounds

118. Which of the following statements concerning use of the short wave diathermy is *incorrect*?

    A.   Induction field heating involves the use of a drum or a cable

    B.   Short wave diathermy is always applied externally, never internally

    C.   Short wave diathermy should not be applied in the near vicinity of a metallic implant

    D.   Electric field heating involves the use of two condenser plates or of pads

119. The single most common problem that may occur with the use of physical agent modalities, resulting in injury to the patient is:

    A.   Skeletal fractures

    B.   Small joint stress fractures

    C.   Avulsion injuries

    D.   Thermal burns

120. Which one of the following statements concerning PAMs is *incorrect*?

    A.   Ultraviolet A and ultraviolet B refer to the use of ultraviolet light therapy

    B.   Intermittent compression is a method of treating lymph edema such as post mastectomy

    C.   Cryotherapy is the therapeutic use of cold

    D.   Ultrasound may be used safely on a patient over an implanted pacemaker

121. One of the statements concerning PAMs is correct. This statement is:

    A.   Paraffin is not inflammable

    B.   The water temperature of a hot pack unit is set at 180° to 185° F

    C.   The hubbard tank is essentially a full-body whirlpool bath

    D.   The inverse square law pertains to the use of the infrared heat lamp

122. One statement concerning the electromyograph (EMG) is *not* true?

    A.   An EMG is a PAM

    B.   The majority of clinical EMGs are done by physiatrists

    C.   Electromyography is based on the principle that electrical currents can be amplified and recorded from contracting muscle tissue

    D.   Correct interpretation of an electromyogram requires training, experience, and practice

123. All the following are types of physical agent modalities still in present usage, *except*:

    A. Massage
    B. Iontophoresis (ion transfer)
    C. Long wave diathermy
    D. Fluidotherapy

124. Therapeutic cold is a modality that in the past has used all of the following; however, there is one agent that is no longer recommended. Which one is it?

    A. Ice massage
    B. Ethyl chloride spray
    C. Fluori-methane spray
    D. Cold packs

125. Erythema "ab igne," or pigmentation, sometimes resulting from prolonged use of infrared radiation, is characterized by:

    A. Dark discoloration with distinct borders
    B. A light uniform red coloration
    C. A homogeneous character
    D. Mottled discoloration

126. A COTA assigned to work with a 25-year-old man whose diagnosis is AIDS should:

    A. Refuse to treat the client
    B. Provide very structured activities
    C. Use universal precautions
    D. Provide progressive strenuous exercises

127. A therapist is performing a MMT, with a shoulder abduction grade of *poor*; what is the patient's body position?

    A. Standing
    B. Supine
    C. Sidelying
    D. Sitting

128. A COTA is observing a patient at bedside and notices that there is no response to painful stimuli. This condition is called:

    A. Stupor
    B. Obtundity
    C. Semicoma
    D. Coma

129. When performing passive ROM, the therapist must consider these objectives, *except*:

    A.   To make the patient aware of desired movements
    B.   To stimulate proprioceptive reflexes involved in joint motion
    C.   To decrease muscle strength
    D.   To attempt to activate the lower motor neuron

130. A therapist is doing a MMT to a patient's shoulder. Horizontal abduction was graded *good*. The client's body position is:

    A.   Supine
    B.   Sitting
    C.   Prone
    D.   Sidelying

131. A COTA is treating a patient who needs muscle reeducation to the right upper extremity. Initially, all of these objectives are of the utmost importance, *except:*

    A.   To develop endurance
    B.   To develop strength
    C.   To develop fine muscle movements
    D.   To develop motor awareness

Part C

Psychosocial Dysfunction

Select the Most Appropriate Answer

1. A 14-year-old girl has been assessed and appears to have a short attention span and difficulty concentrating. The treatment plan will focus first on one of the following:
   A. Assigning the patient an activity that is graded in terms of difficulty to gradually increase her work tolerance
   B. Encouraging the patient to sit for 20-minute periods initially, working on specific tasks
   C. Allowing the patient to work as she pleases and to discontinue the project if she becomes frustrated
   D. Giving the client a book to read on how to increase her attention span

2. When helping plan a general treatment program for a patient with confusion and disorientation, the certified occupational therapy assistant (COTA) should schedule the individual for:
   A. Behavior therapy
   B. Reality orientation
   C. Attitude therapy
   D. Reminiscing therapy

3. When planning a general treatment program for a patient with moderate confusion and decreased interest in the environment, the client should be scheduled for:
   A. Remotivation
   B. Reality orientation
   C. Attitude therapy
   D. Casual conversation with therapist

4. In order to decrease distress of a disoriented client, the COTA should:
   A. Accept the client as he or she is
   B. Decrease distracting stimuli
   C. Encourage decision making
   D. Encourage the client in the performance of creative activities

5. One of the occupational therapy (OT) interventions used for patients with chronic deteriorating conditions is maintaining function as long as possible. Which of the following strategies is recommended in this process?

    A. Encourage personality changes

    B. Try to change the patient's pathology

    C. Deal with the person's assets and ignore his or her liabilities

    D. Enhance the individual's assets and encourage optimum activities

6. A woman client with minimal to moderate socialization skills is going to attend several sessions of a cooperative activity group. The therapist should expect the patient to:

    A. Join the group on her own initiative with active participation

    B. Join the group when asked

    C. Join the group on her own when she wants to, but remain passive

    D. Join the group just to argue with the other members

7. The crucial feature regarding a patient's potential rehabilitative outcome in a psychiatric setting is which of the following?

    A. All team members should work together

    B. The upper rank team member is to indicate what the other members must do

    C. All team members should have therapeutic potential

    D. People with the same diagnosis are treated the same way

8. During the interview process of a client regarding his or her work history, interests, and attitudes, it is strongly recommended to:

    A. Have a list of carefully prepared questions

    B. Ask any question that comes to mind

    C. Ask the client to talk about work in general

    D. Ask questions regarding one of the client's neighbors

9. The first objective for a psychiatric patient who is coming to the OT clinic for the first time is:

    A. To orient him or her to all members of the staff

    B. To "tell" the patient that OT is the best treatment for him or her

    C. To help the patient feel at ease

    D. To introduce him or her to all staff members

10. A 10-year-old child is throwing toys out the window expressing his aggression. Which of the following activities is most appropriate as an OT intervention?

    A. Playing Scrabble®

    B. Reading from a book

    C. Putting a puzzle together

    D. Throwing a bowling ball at pins

11. An 18-year-old man with mental illness who is about to be discharged from the hospital has been referred to OT for prevocational training. This is:

    A. Training for a specific job

    B. Placement in the maintenance department of the hospital

    C. Placement in a nearby hospital

    D. Assessing his work habits, basic skills, and tolerance with the use of simple job tasks

12. A girl with autism who spends most of her time sitting on the floor performing self-abusive activities has been referred to OT. The initial approach should be to:

    A. Perform a formal/informal assessment

    B. Place her in a discussion group

    C. Assign her a simple cleaning job

    D. Give her a ceramic tile project

13. In psychiatric OT clinics, therapists have to be:

    A. Firm with all patients always

    B. Firm with some patients some of the time

    C. Nice with all patients always

    D. Nice only to the patients who follow the rules

14. A man who is pathologically repressing expressions of aggressiveness should use one of the following purposeful activities:

    A. Leather tooling

    B. Weaving on a table loom

    C. A ceramic coil pot

    D. Wedging clay

15. OT intervention for paranoid patients includes:

    A. Activities to decrease egocentricity and allow sublimation of repressed feelings

    B. Activities to divert attention from hallucinations and improve reality testing

    C. Steady quiet activities to reduce motor restlessness

    D. Sedate repetitive activities with little variety

16. There are different roles commonly seen in activity groups used in psychiatric OT clinics. Which of the following statements best describes the role of the "compromiser"?

    A. Nick asks the group if they think T-shirts would sell
    B. Jason admits that maybe some people can't afford to pay $20.00 so he shows his willingness to lower the price to $15.00
    C. Sally wants to use some of the money to help a specific charitable organization
    D. Ginny gets Ralph to explain what is involved in silk-screening

17. When assessing cognitive status, which evaluation would the therapist use?

    A. Map reading
    B. Allen leather lacing evaluation
    C. Fidler diagnostic battery
    D. Goodman battery

18. Jane has just worked through a severe depression and is starting to do some problem solving. In the treatment session, Jane already has identified her problems. What is Jane's next step?

    A. Implementation
    B. Decision making
    C. Identification of alternate solutions
    D. Planning

19. Justin is a 29-year-old man who must learn to concentrate and attend to a task. What performance component would the therapist be working with?

    A. Psychological
    B. Motor
    C. Sensory integration
    D. Cognitive

20. Part of the COTA's job is to observe affect. He or she would be observing:

    A. The degree of worth a person ascribes to himself or herself
    B. An expressed and observed emotion
    C. A process that energizes responses
    D. An investment of emotions in objects

21. Sally is suffering from acute anxiety. What is the COTA's role in helping her to relieve some of the symptoms?

    A. Engage in a constructive activity to occupy the mind
    B. Assist the patient in understanding her assets
    C. Engage in a destructive activity to rid the patient of anger
    D. Engage Sally in an activity that has automatic actions

22. A patient has problems with reality testing. She is schizophrenic and keeps fading into the past and becoming angry. In working a reality testing program, which performance component would you consider?
    A. Cognitive
    B. Motor
    C. Sensory
    D. Psychological

23. Stephen is a drug abuser who has short-term memory deficit. He is being transferred to a halfway house and has to go to the county's assistance office to collect benefits. How can the COTA assist Stephen?
    A. The COTA can take Stephen in his or her car
    B. Schedule sensory integration treatments
    C. Schedule an orientation training session
    D. Schedule group therapy sessions

24. In OT intervention, the assessment part of a depressed person is:
    A. Easy, because the client as a rule is cooperative
    B. Easy, because so much research has been done on the subject
    C. Difficult, because very little research has been done on the subject
    D. Difficult, because the patient has no interest in life

25. Ted is a 7-year-old hyperactive boy with sensory integrative problems. Which of the following types of activities are impractical for him?
    A. Gross motor
    B. Vestibular stimulation
    C. Outcome oriented
    D. Proprioceptive

26. Jane is a 25-year-old woman who displays the following behavior in the OT clinic: acts in a childish fashion, is very dependent on others, and is passive and unmotivated. These signs seem to be due to:
    A. Compensation
    B. Denial
    C. Regression
    D. Depression

27. James is totally irritated that he has to come to OT and does not want anything to do with the therapist. His diagnosis is reactive schizophrenia. The therapist should:

    A.   Sit Jim down and have a long talk about OT and its benefits
    B.   Approach Jim with brief repeated contacts
    C.   Ask Jim to help sweep the clinic to work out his anger
    D.   Give directions and expect an end product by the end of clinic time

28. Choose which activity would be most suitable for an acute schizophrenic just entering the OT clinic:

    A.   Working independently and making a leather wallet with written instructions
    B.   Making a tile trivet with assistance
    C.   Doing peacock loom—patchwork pattern
    D.   Tailoring a suit

29. When providing for self-concept development and sense of personal worth, choose the best activity:

    A.   Arranging a party
    B.   Building a bird house—woodworking
    C.   Sanding blocks for preschool class
    D.   Engraving one's initials on a leather project

30. Reality testing is often necessary for realistic concepts about the environment. Choose the best program or activity to use for this:

    A.   Plaster of paris free carving
    B.   Copying a charcoal design
    C.   Making an unstructured tile mosaic
    D.   Using clay free form

31. Tom enters the OT clinic very quietly and sits in the far corner. Which of the following would you *not* do?

    A.   Tell him how well he will do and how much better he will feel if he joins the group
    B.   Approach slowly
    C.   Eliminate the need to make a decision
    D.   Be cautious in giving praise

32. Which of the following would the therapist expect to see in a depressed patient?

    A.   Cooperation
    B.   Adjustment to the facility
    C.   Disagreement with OT treatment
    D.   Suppression of anger

33. A COTA has a group of patients, several of which are depressed and new to the clinic. Which of the following activities would best suit this beginning group?

    A. Planning a spaghetti dinner for the whole ward
    B. Building a booth for the forthcoming fair
    C. Putting on a fashion show
    D. Copying a simple colored paper collage for the hallway

34. When treating the manic patient, which of the following would *not* be taken into consideration?

    A. Activities that require very little energy
    B. Activities that require a moderate amount of physical exertion
    C. Activities that give a feeling of accomplishment
    D. Activities that give an outlet for hostility

35. In OT intervention, which of the following is therapeutic for the obsessive-compulsive person?

    A. Activities of a low concentration level that offer immediate gratification
    B. Activities that do not require decision making
    C. Activities that the client can control and that enable him or her to make decisions
    D. Activities that involve repetitive movements and have clear instructions

36. Sam is a patient who just entered the OT clinic and, upon evaluation, had the following problems identified: negative self-image, fear of being followed, and sexual inhibitions and disturbances. Which of Maslow's hierarchy of needs must be taken into consideration in current treatment?

    A. Safety
    B. Cognitive
    C. Self-esteem
    D. Physiological
    E. A, C, and D

37. A therapist is using reality therapy with a patient through a task group. Which of the following would be appropriate in this type of approach?

    A. Praise the client when he makes mistakes for trying his best
    B. The patient acts out and the therapist places him in a time-out chair
    C. Use "day dreaming" techniques
    D. The client has worked only 3 days; the therapist, in conjunction with the patient, decides to increase his attendance to 6 days

38. This OT clinic uses client-centered therapy. Which of the following is/are appropriate steps of approach?

    A. View the world through the eyes of the other individual
    B. Accept all the different behaviors exhibited by the person
    C. Maintain honesty in the relationship with the client
    D. All the above

39. The Model of Human Occupation includes all of the following levels of internal organization except:

    A. Performance
    B. Volition
    C. Obsession
    D. Aged

40. John is a schizophrenic on Haldol and Cogentin. Which one of the following would the therapist *not* want to do?

    A. Administer activities that avoid gross motor actions to reduce sudden movements
    B. Keep the patient in the shade if doing activities outside
    C. Suggest activities that allow for sudden postural changes
    D. Allow the patient to get water whenever he needs it

41. Jane is a manic who is now medicated and doing well. She has just started in the OT clinic. Which of the possible side effects would the therapist be most concerned about?

    A. Confusion with slurred speech
    B. Photosensitivity
    C. Flight of ideas
    D. Inactivity

42. Sam is severely depressed and has just come for treatment. He is placed on a tricyclic drug (Sinequan) and enters therapy. Which *one* of the following is pertinent?

    A. Sam may have seizures but he will have immediate relief from his depression
    B. Sam's tremors are problematic and he will have continuous weight loss
    C. Sam may be a suicide risk for some time even though he is now on medication
    D. Sam may have to use Artane with Sinequan to control the drowsiness

43. Sally has frequent anxiety attacks and has started using Xanax. Which *one* of the following would you consider when programming?

    A. The patient may have drowsiness, light-headedness, or adverse behavioral affects
    B. The patient needs to engage in activities such as tatting or card weaving
    C. The patient may choose woodworking that would include use of the band saw
    D. The patient will be able to organize well and have a high energy level

44. Claire is a new patient in the OT clinic. She is schizophrenic and is somewhat regressed. Which of the following is correct?

    A. Foster security in the treatment setting by allowing a dependency relationship
    B. The patient must be met at a moderate to fast volitional level
    C. She has a right to attention, approval, and suicide
    D. You must use an expectant attitude to gain results

45. Mary is a 67-year-old woman who has been in a state hospital for 10 years. She is diagnosed as schizophrenic and has very little contact with reality. You must prove that reality can be rewarding. Which of the following would you use?

    A. Be sensitive to present needs and wants
    B. Acknowledge fears and anxieties
    C. Give sufficient support to ensure feelings of success
    D. Locate a separate place of treatment for a testing environment
    E. All the above

46. Chronic schizophrenic patients were placed in a resocialization program for 3 months, and then transferred to foster care. Significant improvement was noticed in one of the following areas:

    A. Speech
    B. Safety precautions
    C. Social interest and competence
    D. Personal grooming

47. Jody is a multiply handicapped individual with hallucinations. She requires activities that give reality contact. Choose one of the following:

    A. Acrylic painting on canvas
    B. Leather lacing
    C. Clay—free form
    D. Carving plaster of paris

48. Kathy is a woman with schizophrenia who has come to the stage of centering on the development of self-concept, ego strength, and sense of personal worth. Which of the following would be the best for her?

    A. Block printing stationery with her initial
    B. Sewing a new skirt—easy pattern
    C. Stringing a new necklace
    D. Using a floor loom with an intricate pattern

49. The schizophrenic needs an opportunity to improve sensory perception. Which of the following is *not* included in this area?

    A. Rhythms—clapping, stamping
    B. Bright colors
    C. Coloring books
    D. Stuffed toys

50. A group of young adults in a halfway house situation are meeting in the evening to discuss self-concept and the process of change. Which of the topics should be included in this discussion?

    A. Will to change
    B. Skill to change
    C. Time of day activities
    D. Realistic expectations
    E. A and D
    F. B and C

51. The COTA is observing a group of regressed patients with schizophrenia. Many of these persons communicate nonverbally. What area(s) would the therapist observe to help understand the messages being given?

    A. Gestures
    B. Lighting in the room
    C. Furniture
    D. Posture
    E. A and D
    F. B and D

52. An 80-year-old woman shows marked changes in judgment, memory, orientation, labile affect, comprehension, and regression. With these symptoms, the therapist may identify one of the following:

    A. Depression
    B. Organic brain syndrome
    C. Schizophrenia—catatonic state
    D. Schizophrenia—paranoid state

53. Tom, who displays poor self-identification, distrust, suspicion, hostility, superior attitude, delusions of grandeur, and persecution appears to:

    A. Be a schizophrenic—paranoid type
    B. Be a schizophrenic—catatonic type
    C. Have an antisocial personality
    D. Have an organic brain syndrome

54. The process of selecting treatment methods in a psychiatric setting includes all of the following areas except:

    A. Therapeutic approach
    B. Activities
    C. Diagnoses
    D. Environment

55. Nancy presents the following symptoms in an OT clinic: loss of self-esteem, loneliness, fear, introjected hostility, hallucinations, delusions, poor ego boundaries, poor socialization, withdrawal, and regression. Upon observation of Nancy's behavior, the therapist seems to think that this client had one of the following conditions:

    A. Schizophrenia—catatonic type
    B. Obsessive compulsive personality
    C. Schizophrenia—paranoid type
    D. Schizophrenia—hebephrenic type

56. Which of the following is *not* a category of OT intervention?

    A. Functional restoration
    B. Psychopharmacology
    C. Prevention
    D. Maintenance of function

57. Miss J. is a 65-year-old woman who has been diagnosed with dementia. Her symptoms affect her social and occupational performance. Which of the following is appropriate for Miss J?

    A. Provide an unstructured "milieu"
    B. Provide an unfamiliar environment
    C. Provide frequent contact with nonstressful familiar objects
    D. Provide conversation with diversified content

58. One of the methods commonly used in psychiatric treatment is problem solving. This basically means:

    A. Identification of the problem, generation and evaluation of possible solutions
    B. Preference of not acknowledging the problem
    C. After acknowledging the problem, the client is undecided regarding the most appropriate solution to explore
    D. After acknowledging the problem, there is no generation of possible solutions

59. Tom is a 15-year-old boy with a borderline personality disorder who was referred to the OT clinic. Upon evaluation, the therapist developed a treatment plan and implemented, through activities, one of the following:

    A. Unstructured and stressful situations
    B. Exciting experiences
    C. Clear, prompt, and consistent limits
    D. Unreliable relationships with staff members

60. Persons with obsessive-compulsive disorders should perform one of the following:

    A. Activities that they can control and that encourage decision making
    B. Activities that require little concentration and offer moderate gratification
    C. Activities that are structured and provide repetitive movements
    D. Activities that are unstructured and provide a diversified amount of movements

61. A mute catatonic woman is in the OT clinic folding bandages. Suddenly, this client, upon the folding process, starts to put the bandages in her mouth. The therapist should:

    A. Immediately stop her and give her another project
    B. Ignore her actions
    C. Scold the patient
    D. Offer her something to eat

62. Kim, a 14-year-old girl who is angry and acting-out, was referred to OT. Upon evaluation, she was placed in a structured group with strict rules. This treatment approach in psychiatry is termed:

    A. Progressive therapy
    B. Directive or repressive
    C. Behavior therapy
    D. Psychoanalytic

63. Irene, a 16-year-old girl, was assigned to work in a group with other clients who were making their own projects. The therapist gave a ball of clay to Irene, who told the therapist that she was depressed and therefore unable to work with ceramics. One ½ hour later, the therapist checked the patient and saw that the sculpture of a man sitting on a rock, called *The Thinker*, had emerged. During the performance of this purposeful activity, the patient was working in what type of group:

    A. Project group
    B. Egocentric cooperative group
    C. Rationalization group
    D. Parallel group

64. In supportive therapy, which is an approach used in psychiatric OT clinics, the therapist should:

    A. Communicate with the patient casually
    B. Enhance the patient's assets
    C. Enhance the patient's liabilities
    D. It does not matter so long as an approach is made

65. During the evaluation process of an individual with a psychosocial dysfunction, the therapist asks the patient to perform a simple activity with few instructions. The therapist appears to be testing which of the following?

    A. Work tolerance
    B. Cognition
    C. Manual dexterity
    D. Strength

66. The therapeutic approach aspect of selecting treatment must consider all of the following except:

    A. Motivation
    B. The therapist's preference
    C. Values
    D. Learning styles

67. A therapist analyzed a specific activity and gave it to a psychiatric patient with the purpose of developing competence and balance within the patient's interaction with society. This type of analysis is termed:

   A. Biomechanical
   B. Occupational behavior
   C. Neurodevelopmental
   D. Sensory integrative

68. B.J. is a woman who works in a group at the OT clinic participating in assembly line ceramics by glazing bisque. She claims that she comes to OT just because her doctor wants her to. During the performance of the activity, lack of interest is shown by arriving systematically late to the OT sessions and having frequent accidents, such as dropping jars of glaze. One of the following is the recommended method to deal with B.J.:

   A. Refuse her participation in the group because of the disruptive behavior
   B. Give her another type of activity
   C. Set up specific expectations and meet with her periodically to discuss her behavioral performance
   D. Allow her to gain more control within the group

69. A group of patients in the OT clinic is working on collages. One patient uses only one picture on his or her project. The therapist may conclude that this patient most likely is diagnosed as:

   A. Compulsive
   B. Obsessive
   C. Depressed
   D. Having a personality disorder

70. A patient in the OT clinic is painting using heavy strokes. This may be a sign of:

   A. Fear
   B. Self-assertiveness
   C. Unassertiveness
   D. Instability

71. An adolescent in the OT clinic is drawing with extreme symmetry and perfection. This type of behavior may be an indication of:

    A. Rationalization
    B. Insecurity
    C. Assertiveness
    D. Rigidity and compulsiveness

72. A group of patients is working on the monthly ward calendar, under the supervision of a COTA. This activity is an example of which type of group?

    A. Egocentric
    B. Cooperative
    C. Project
    D. Immature

73. A patient who is uncooperative, refuses treatment for his or her condition, and is unwilling to take care of his or her own health is exhibiting one of the following:

    A. Anger
    B. Anxiety
    C. Repression
    D. Negative denial

74. A patient exhibiting depression, withdrawal, aggressiveness, and acting-out behavior in the OT department is using one of the following mechanisms:

    A. Regression
    B. Anger
    C. Repression
    D. Positive denial

75. A woman diagnosed with anorexia nervosa exhibits the following symptoms: abnormal eating habits, improper nutrition, excessive physical exercise, and the inability to identify and verbalize internal states. Which of the following is/are appropriate for this client:

    A. Provide activities for self-expression
    B. Provide activities for self-experimentation
    C. Provide a structured environment with a balanced routine of daily activities
    D. All the above

76. A COTA is leading a group of clients performing individual activities. One of the patients has an epileptic seizure. The therapist should:
    A. Place the client sidelying
    B. Loosen any restraints of clothing
    C. Ask the other patients to leave the room
    D. Call a nurse immediately
    E. A and B
    F. C and D

77. When interviewing a patient, the therapist should:
    A. Ask questions that lead to one- or two-word answers
    B. Ignore any questions asked by the client
    C. Ask questions that do not lead to one- or two-word answers
    D. Talk more than the client

78. A therapist, whose role is defined as a rehabilitator in the mental health field, must consider the following objectives *except*:
    A. To assess a patient's condition and make recommendations
    B. To teach appropriate interpersonal relationships
    C. To encourage dependency
    D. To reinforce stress management techniques

79. When the occupational therapist works with clients who are chemically dependent, he or she must set the following objectives, *except:*
    A. To evaluate work performance
    B. To ignore a patient's symptoms
    C. To prepare the client to return to the work force
    D. To encourage participation in support groups

Answer Key

Section IV
Occupational Therapy Intervention—Part A

Pediatrics

1. C. Chaining. **2.** C. Instructions should be detailed and long. **3.** D. All the above. **4.** B. Crocheting. **5.** B. The construction and supervision of the use of orthoses. **6.** A. A child has poor head and trunk control. **7.** B. Directionality. **8.** B. Motor planning. **9.** D. The Bruininks-Oseretsky Motor Developmental Scale. **10.** C. Dressing skills.

11. C. Games with one other person. **12.** D. Hanging string art on the wall. **13.** D. Copy a square, circle, and triangle. **14.** E. Rood approach. **15.** C. Equilibrium reactions. **16.** C. Three-point pinch. **17.** C. Dress up. **18.** C. To delay the development of deformities. **19.** E. All the above. **20.** C. Bed and wheelchair activities.

21. A. The flexion of the arm and leg on the skull side and/or an increase in flexor tone, and the extension of the arm and leg on the face side and/or an increase in extensor tone. **22.** D. Associated reactions. **23.** A. The body rotates as a whole in the same direction. **24.** B. Minimal or no further recovery is expected. **25.** C. 4 years of age. **26.** A. Laterality. **27.** C. He or she mirrored every activity. **28.** B. A diagonal line. **29.** D. Both B) A count the dot test and C) Picking out a specific number from a line of random numbers. **30.** C. Distinguish the difference between 1 lb and 3 lb sand bags.

31. A. Has problems with laterality. **32.** D. All the above. **33.** C. Use a multisensory stimulation approach. **34.** E. Answers A) Tactile stimuli, B) Visual stimuli and D) Olfactory stimuli. **35.** B. He or she draws a circle toward the dominant side. **36.** C. To obtain 120° of shoulder flexion. **37.** E. All the above. **38.** A. Sensory integrative disorder. **39.** C. Rolling from one side to the other in bed. **40.** C. The child and the play guide the therapy.

41. D. All the above. **42.** B. The thumb in front of the chin, the middle finger under the chin, the index finger on the side of the cheek. **43.** A. Does the child maintain his or her head erect in the midline during writing? **44.** D. A hearing aid. **45.** C. To encourage dependency in dressing skills to prevent further muscle weakness. **46.** B. Magazine picture collages. **47.** D. Desensitization techniques. **48.** A. Touch the body parts to be moved. **49.** C. Perception. **50.** D. Stereognosis.

51. B. Normal development occurs from a lateral direction to a medial direction. **52.** A. Antigravity exercises. **53.** B. A glove puppet. **54.** B. Body scheme. **55.** C. Spatial relations. **56.** D. Both A) Biomechanical and B) Neurodevelopmental. **57.** B. Sensory integrative. **58.** B. Increasing the child's reach. **59.** A. Flexors. **60.** C. Inclined upwards.

61. B. The identification of position change of body parts, without visual cues when performed by someone other than the patient. **62.** B. Riding a scooter board in a prone position. **63.** A. Isolate each of the various steps of the activity. **64.** E. All the above. **65.** A. Colorful, large, three-dimensional toys. **66.** B. A scooter board. **67.** C. Rattles of various shapes and colors. **68.** B. Blocks. **69.** A. Projective technique. **70.** D. Demanding increased sensory image and discrimination.

71. B. Goals that are realistic given the level of retardation. **72.** A. Front-opening garments.

Part B

Physical Dysfunction

1. F. All the above. **2.** B. An interest questionnaire. **3.** D. All the above. **4.** C. Sustained positions of the hand. **5.** B. A tile trivet. **6.** A. Respiratory dysfunctions. **7.** D. Isolate the individual steps of the activity. **8.** D. All the above. **9.** A. Remove the footrest from the uninvolved side and begin with the patient using both unaffected extremities. **10.** A. To incorporate the new limb substitute within his or her body's schema.

11. A. Put the garment on the amputated side first. **12.** D. Both A) Use one-handed pots and pans and C) Examine oneself for burns because of diminished sensation of the involved upper extremity. **13.** B. Device forcing fingers toward radial deviation. **14.** C. The uninvolved leg and uninvolved arm. **15.** A. Put the involved arm into the sleeve first. **16.** B. Remove the uninvolved arm first. **17.** A. Hold the load as close to the body as possible. **18.** A. Maintaining the range of wrist extension and forearm supination. **19.** A. Use a straight-back chair inside the bathtub. **20.** D. Review the patient's chart for updating information before proceeding.

21. A. Bowl stabilizer. **22.** A. Work habits, manual dexterity, and endurance. **23.** C. Identify the techniques and their steps, and practice each activity repeatedly. **24.** A. Give patients leisure opportunities. **25.** C. Immediately be encouraged to use the involved side for feeding, toileting, transferring, etc. **26.** C. A shopping cart. **27.** C. Signs of fatigue. **28.** B. Practicing going up and down the steps. **29.** B. Side by side. **30.** A. Use one hand rather than two.

31. A. Lift all pans and other objects as opposed to sliding them. **32.** B. Allow the patient to rest briefly and observe the signs. **33.** C. Radial. **34.** C. Engage in meaningful conversation. **35.** D. Explain in detail one's own background, school attended, marital status, age, etc. **36.** A. While the patient is still in bed. **37.** D. External power. **38.** D. All the above. **39.** C. Gravity. **40.** C. Lock the wheels of the wheelchair.

41. C. Decrease stiffness and increase ROM. **42.** C. Partially sponge bathe herself without assistance. **43.** C. Observe for any possible physical discomfort. **44.** C. Break down the activity into smaller steps. **45.** D. Work habits. **46.** C. The latissimus dorsi. **47.** C. Roll in bed from side to side. **48.** C. Suspended on a deltoid aid (overhead arm sling). **49.** B. Time and energy conservation techniques. **50.** B. The patient's motivation to become independent.

51. B. Use heavy pots and pans in the kitchen to decrease tremors. **52.** C. Radial nerve. **53.** A. Using a wheelchair with an opening back rest, approach the back of the wheelchair to the front of the toilet seat, lock the wheelchair, and slide back using push-ups. **54.** B. Active exercises several times a day. **55.** D. Both A) Rigidity and C) Bradykinesia. **56.** D. All the above. **57.** A. A standard wheelchair. **58.** A. Tilt the patient back, and elevate his legs. **59.** D. Not permit the wrist to be positioned in extreme flexion. **60.** D. Use the affected hand as a helper.

61. C. Has completed use training. **62.** D. Necessary activities to maintain life support needs. **63.** C. New patterns of life need to be initiated. **64.** B. Hydraulic lift transfer. **65.** B. Sliding board transfer. **66.** D. Patient and family. **67.** B. Perception. **68.** D. All the above. **69.** D. All the above. **70.** C. Energy conservation.

71. B. Joint protection. **72.** B. Neurodevelopmental. **73.** A. Antigravity exercises. **74.** C. The maximal resistance the patient is able to sustain and overcome successfully. **75.** C. Spasticity on the involved side. **76.** B. Limitation of the fingers at the MCPJs is present. **77.** A. Improve strength to fair (3). **78.** D. Therapist and patient. **79.** B. Work hardening. **80.** A. Self-care.

81. A. The involved side. **82.** B. Activities that maintain a specific position for a prolonged period of time. **83.** B. The edema stage is in progress. **84.** C. Amputation—preprosthetic evaluation—preprosthetic treatment (when necessary)—prescription—fabrication—initial checkout—training—final checkout. **85.** A. Open/close terminal device (TD). **86.** D. Opening of the TD. **87.** D. The day of admission. **88.** C. Before the patient begins use training. **89.** B. A conservative treatment in LBP. **90.** A. Knitting.

91. C. A person's body. **92.** A. Gather, analyze, and interpret pertinent information. **93.** D. Reevaluate the splint to ensure less pressure in the area that produced redness. **94.** B. Report the situation to the supervisor. **95.** A. On the dominant side of the brain. **96.** C. Hand and fingers. **97.** D. Patients with quadriplegia and older patients with poliomyelitis. **98.** B. There is limitation in extension of the elbow joint. **99.** C. Rehabilitative. **100.** C. Sitting and performing table activities.

101. B. Muscle weakness. **102.** C. Ulnar nerve. **103.** B. Approximately 30° in dorsiflexion. **104.** C. Distal palmar crease. **105.** B. Grades of manual muscle testing. **106.** A. Prevention of soft tissue contractures. **107.** B. Ultraviolet light. **108.** D. Paraffin dip. **109.** D. Higher tissue temperatures can be maintained than with the use of other modalities. **110.** C. Low voltage galvanic (direct) current.

111. B. Patient comfort is unreliable, as to dosage intensity of ultrasound. **112.** D. Ultrasonic diathermy and short wave diathermy are essentially similar. **113.** B. With normal circulation and sensation, the danger of overheating is minimal. **114.** B. The patient's marital status. **115.** C. There is evidence of muscle contraction, but no joint motion is detected. **116.** A. Peripheral vascular disease. **117.** D. Open wounds. **118.** B. Short wave diathermy is always applied externally, never internally. **119.** D. Thermal burns. **120.** D. Ultrasound may be used safely on a patient over an implanted pacemaker.

121. C. The hubbard tank is essentially a full-body whirlpool bath. **122.** A. An EMG is a PAM. **123.** C. Long wave diathermy. **124.** B. Ethyl chloride spray. **125.** D. Mottled discoloration. **126.** C. Use universal precautions. **127.** B. Supine. **128.** D. Coma. **129.** C. To decrease muscle strength. **130.** B. Sitting.

131. C. To develop fine muscle movements.

Part C

Psychosocial Dysfunction

1. A. Assigning the patient an activity that is graded in terms of difficulty to gradually increase her work tolerance. **2.** B. Reality orientation. **3.** A. Remotivation. **4.** B. Decrease distracting stimuli. **5.** D. Enhance the individual's assets and encourage optimum activities. **6.** B. Join the group when asked. **7.** A. All team members should work together. **8.** A. Have a list of carefully prepared questions. **9.** C. To help the patient feel at ease. **10.** D. Throwing a bowling ball at the pins.

11. D. Assessing his work habits, basic skills, and tolerance with the use of simple job tasks. **12.** A. Perform a formal/informal assessment. **13.** B. Firm with some patients some of the time. **14.** D. Wedging clay. **15.** B. Activities to divert attention from hallucinations and improve reality testing. **16.** B. Jason admits that maybe some people can't afford to pay $20.00 so he shows his willingness to lower the price to $15.00. **17.** B. Allen leather lacing evaluation. **18.** C. Identification of alternate solutions. **19.** D. Cognitive. **20.** B. An expressed and observed emotion.

21. A. Engage in a constructive activity to occupy the mind. **22.** D. Psychological. **23.** C. Schedule an orientation training session. **24.** D. Difficult, because the patient has no interest in life. **25.** C. Outcome oriented. **26.** C. Regression. **27.** B. Approach Jim with brief repeated contacts. **28.** B. Making a tile trivet with assistance. **29.** D. Engraving one's initials on a leather project. **30.** B. Copying a charcoal design.

31. A. Tell him how well he will do and how much better he will feel if he joins the group. **32.** C. Disagreement with OT treatment. **33.** D. Copying a simple colored paper collage for the hallway. **34.** A. Activities that require very little energy. **35.** D. Activities that involve repetitive movements and have clear instructions. **36.** E. Answers A) Safety, C) Self-esteem and D) Physiological. **37.** D. The client has worked only 3 days; the therapist, in conjunction with the patient, decides to increase attendance to 6 days. **38.** D. All the above. **39.** C. Obsession. **40.** C. Suggest activities that allow for sudden postural changes.

41. C. Flight of ideas. **42.** C. Sam may be a suicide risk for some time even though he is now on medication. **43.** A. The patient may have drowsiness, light-headedness, or adverse behavioral effects. **44.** D. You must use an expectant attitude to gain results. **45.** B. Acknowledge fears and anxieties. **46.** C. Social interest and competence. **47.** B. Leather lacing. **48.** A. Block printing stationery with her initial. **49.** D. Stuffed toys. **50.** E. Both A) Will to change and D) Realistic expectations.

51. E. Both A) Gestures and D) Posture. **52.** B. Organic brain syndrome. **53.** A. Be a schizophrenic—paranoid type. **54.** C. Diagnoses. **55.** A. Schizophrenia—catatonic type. **56.** B. Psychopharmacology. **57.** C. Provide frequent contact with nonstressful familiar objects. **58.** A. Identification of the problem, generation and evaluation of possible solutions. **59.** C. Clear, prompt, and consistent limits. **60.** C. Activities that are structured and provide repetitive movements.

61. A. Immediately stop her and give her another project. **62.** B. Directive or repressive. **63.** D. Parallel group. **64.** B. Enhance the patient's assets. **65.** B. Cognition. **66.** B. The therapist's preference. **67.** B. Occupational behavior. **68.** C. Set up specific expectations and meet with her periodically to discuss her behavioral performance. **69.** A. Compulsive. **70.** B. Self-assertiveness.

71. D. Rigidity and compulsiveness. **72.** C. Project. **73.** D. Negative denial. **74.** B. Anger. **75.** D. All the above. **76.** E. Both A) Place the client sidelying and B) Loosen any restraints of clothing. **77.** C. Ask questions that do not lead to one- or two-word answers. **78.** C. To encourage dependency. **79.** B. To ignore a patient's symptoms.

SECTION V

Ethics and Fieldwork

General Fieldwork Information

When making ethical decisions and deciding on your best course of action when presented with an ethical decision, there are several factors you must take into consideration. It is important you be aware of general ethical principles, legal considerations, and the rules and guidelines that govern our profession. The following questions have been designed to increase your awareness of these factors. Some general questions that you may want to ask yourself when facing an ethical decision are:

1. Who does it harm or benefit? Does it deny anyone's rights? Does it protect anyone's rights?
2. What legal issues are involved? What laws govern this situation? What public or private agencies are involved?
3. Does it meet established codes and standards for the profession?
4. What would other therapists do in a similar situation?
5. Could I reveal my decision openly to others?

General Ethical Principles

1. Beneficence can be defined as:
   A. The obligation to help others
   B. The principle of maintaining a patient's privacy
   C. A patient's right to make his or her own decisions
   D. The obligation that we should maintain agreements made with a patient

2. Veracity can be defined as:
   A. A relationship between the practitioner and a patient whereby both are bound to the truth
   B. The right of the practitioner to provide care for the patient without the patient's informed consent
   C. The patient's right to make his or her own decisions
   D. The belief that the practitioner can make decisions for the patient if the outcome of the action is good

3. Nonmaleficence can be defined as:

   A. "Above all, do no harm"
   B. The basic principle that deals with fairness
   C. The principle that requires action within the professional standards of practice
   D. "Do unto others as you would have them do unto you"

4. Autonomy can be defined as:

   A. The patient's right to participate in and decide on healthcare decisions
   B. Following your own moral principles as a practitioner
   C. Being impartial in making ethical decisions
   D. Maintaining professional competence

5. The "Reasonably Prudent Man" theory can be defined as:

   A. Making informed consent decisions
   B. Using the most cost effective means to an end
   C. Using time effectively
   D. Acting in a way that other practitioners would, in a similar situation, without benefit of hindsight or foresight

6. The branch of ethics known as *deontology* can be described as:

   A. A study of morals
   B. Allowing the consequences or outcome to dictate our actions
   C. Doing one's duty despite the outcome or consequences
   D. A study of values

7. The branch of ethics known as *teleology* can be described as:

   A. Making decisions based on religious morals
   B. Making decisions based on the outcomes and consequences relating to those involved as opposed to simply doing one's duty
   C. Doing one's duty despite the outcome
   D. Making decisions based on the majority of media influence

Application of General Ethical Principles

8. The best example of beneficence is:
   A. The decision to shorten a therapy session despite a company mandate to provide full sessions for each patient because a patient is complaining of pain
   B. The decision to visit a patient on your day off because you promised to do so
   C. The decision to respect the right of a patient to refuse therapy despite the fact that therapy will help the patient
   D. The decision to keep information confidential about a patient when asked by a family member

9. The best example of veracity is:
   A. The decision to shorten a therapy session despite a company mandate to provide full sessions for each patient because a patient is complaining of pain
   B. The decision to visit a patient on your day off because you promised to do so
   C. The decision to respect the right of a patient to refuse therapy despite the fact that therapy will help the patient
   D. The decision to keep information confidential about a patient when asked by a family member

10. The best example of nonmaleficence is:
    A. The decision to refuse to do minimal assist transfers with a patient who has poor sitting balance when requested by your supervisor
    B. The decision to shorten a therapy session despite a company mandate to provide full sessions for each patient because a patient is complaining of pain
    C. The decision to visit a patient on your day off because you promised to do so
    D. The decision to respect the right of a patient to refuse therapy despite the fact that therapy will help the patient

11. When problems arise in fieldwork, the first thing to do is:
    A. Talk with the fieldwork coordinator
    B. Talk with the supervisor
    C. Discuss the issue with other fieldwork students
    D. Call your parents

12. You are a Level II Fieldwork student in a geriatric facility. Your assigned client, Mrs. Smith, is a 90-year-old woman who has been diagnosed with left hemiplegia and is oriented to time, place, and person. Mrs. Smith refuses to attend therapy and states, "OT won't make me any better." Your best course of action to take next is:

    A. Let Mrs. Smith stay in her room because she has a right to refuse therapy
    B. Talk with Mrs. Smith about potential outcomes of therapy
    C. Let Mrs. Smith stay in her room because she is old and you do not want to cause her to suffer
    D. Tell Mrs. Smith you are taking her for a walk and then stop in the occupational therapy (OT) clinic for therapy

13. Your fieldwork supervisor asks you not to tell your patients that you are a fieldwork student because some of them may not want to be treated by a student. The first thing you should so is:

    A. Report your supervisor to the American Occupational Therapy Association (AOTA) for a violation of professional ethics
    B. Tell your supervisor that you must accurately represent your competence and training
    C. Tell your supervisor, "okay" but represent yourself as a student to the patients
    D. Comply with the supervisor's request unless a patient specifically asks you if you are a student

14. The policy of your fieldwork facility states, "The student supervisor is permitted to claim any treatment units performed by the student only if the supervisor is on-site during treatment." You notice that your supervisor has been claiming treatment units when he or she was not physically present with you during treatment. You decide to report the supervisor to the AOTA for making fraudulent claims, which one of the following is true?

    A. No violation of professional ethics has occurred
    B. Your supervisor has acted unethically
    C. The student has acted unethically
    D. Both the student and supervisor have acted unethically

15. You are a fieldwork student in an extended care facility. You notice that incontinent patients do not have their incontinent pads changed immediately. You believe that the patients are not being cared for properly. Your best course of action to take is to:

    A. Discuss the situation with your supervisor to find out the facility's policy on this
    B. Wait until the completion of your fieldwork and then file a complaint with Medicare
    C. Tell the certified nursing assistant (CNA) that patients should have their pads changed immediately
    D. Change the pads for patients if you notice they are wet

16. During fieldwork, you are assigned a patient diagnosed with AIDS. It is ethically possible to refuse to treat this patient if:

    A. It is against your religious beliefs
    B. You believe it is morally correct to do so
    C. You have a medical condition that may endanger the patient
    D. Your supervisor agrees with your decision

17. Mr. James is a patient diagnosed in the early stages of terminal cancer. He requests that his wife not be told because she would "just worry." Because Mr. James has been assigned as your patient, his wife asks you how soon her husband will "get better." In deciding whether or not to tell Mr. James' wife the truth, which one of the following considerations is true in this situation?

    A. Your primary ethical duty is to the wife
    B. Your primary ethical duty is to Mr. James
    C. The wife's "right to know" is an ethical and legal right
    D. Your ethical duty is to both Mr. James and his wife

18. Evelyn is a patient diagnosed with a brain injury following a car accident. After a fall in her apartment, she enters rehabilitation for activities of daily living (ADL) training. She is a heavy smoker and states that she has always enjoyed only "smoking and listening to music." You have decided that in order to treat Evelyn holistically, you will "keep after" her to develop a healthy lifestyle and quit smoking. Your supervisor tells you that you actions are a violation of Evelyn's personal rights. Which one of the following is true?

    A. Evelyn has a right to decide and pursue her own enjoyments even if her habits are unhealthy
    B. Because Evelyn has a brain injury, you have an obligation to make healthy decisions for her
    C. Evelyn's need for a healthy lifestyle outweighs her need for pleasure, so your decision was ethically correct
    D. Your decision is ethically correct because the good (i.e., she might quit smoking) outweighs the bad (i.e., "keeping after" her)

19. As a Fieldwork Level II student, you have been assigned to Mrs. Wareham, who needs assistance for training in self-feeding skills. You begin treatment, then realize that you are running behind schedule. You feed Mrs. Wareham because it is quicker and justify your actions because she was feeling tired anyway, Which one of the following is true?

    A. You have violated your agreement to treat Mrs. Wareham
    B. You are ethically correct because your actions were driven by kindness toward the patient
    C. You have violated Mrs. Wareham's right to participate in treatment
    D. You are ethically correct because the end justifies the means

20. Mrs. Holtz is an 80-year-old patient assigned to you during your Fieldwork II. She is frail and is restrained in a wheelchair. As you pass her in the hallway, Mrs. Holtz calls out and complains, "Please take me for a walk. I get so tired from sitting all the time." What should you do?

    A. Remove her restraint and take her for a walk
    B. Tell Mrs. Holtz that you are not allowed to walk patients
    C. Report the situation to the nurse
    D. Ask the CNA for permission to walk with Mrs. Holtz

21. Mrs. Lidwell, a 40-year-old woman, was diagnosed with a cerebrovascular accident (CVA) following the birth of her child. Mrs. Lidwell is motivated to gain complete recovery of her right upper extremity but the physician believes that Mrs. Lidwell will have permanent severe impairments. Mrs. Lidwell, who is in outpatient rehabilitation, spends all of her time working toward increased function. You feel it is your duty to be honest, so, when Mrs. Lidwell asks you if she will recover completely, you truthfully answer, "no." Mrs. Lidwell refuses further therapy. Your supervisor tells you that you have harmed this patient. Who is ethically correct, you or your supervisor?

    A. Your supervisor is correct because you were beneficent
    B. Your supervisor is correct because you failed to identify that Mrs. Lidwell's motivation was the largest contributing factor to any potential recovery, and may have taken away any chance for recovery
    C. You are correct because you should always be honest with patients
    D. You are correct because Mrs. Lidwell has a right to informed consent

Legal Considerations

22. Title VII of the Civil Rights Act of 1964 provides protection for a student based on:

    A. Sex
    B. Handicap
    C. Age
    D. Race

23. The Family Educational Rights and Privacy Act is also known as:

    A. The Buckley Amendment
    B. Section 504
    C. IDEA
    D. Title IX

24. The Family Educational Rights and Privacy Act provides a student protection concerning:

    A. Private notes and materials maintained by instructors
    B. Only information contained in school records
    C. Access and disclosure of information about a student
    D. Only disability information

Application of Legal Considerations

25. The Fieldwork Coordinator obtains a signed release from a student requesting permission to release information on the student's previous fieldwork performance. This is an example of the requirements of:

    A. The Buckley Amendment
    B. Section 504
    C. Title IX
    D. Title VII

26. An example of information *not* available to the student under the provisions of the Buckley Amendment include:

    A. Official records maintained by the fieldwork site
    B. Medical, psychiatric, and counseling records
    C. Letters of reference completed by the fieldwork site
    D. Letters of reference provided by the academic program

27. Section 504 of the Rehabilitation Act of 1973 provides protection for a student with a disability access to the same educational opportunities as other persons. The best example of "reasonable accommodation" for a student with a disability is:

    A. A student with fine motor problems is permitted to dictate progress notes
    B. Transfers, which are considered an essential job function at this facility, are omitted as a fieldwork objective for the student with a wheelchair
    C. The student with Attention Deficit Disorder is not required to complete the comprehensive case study required for all students
    D. The student with short-term memory problems is permitted to audiotape interviews with all clients

28. According to the intent of Section 504, in the evaluation of a student with a disability, the fieldwork educator should:
    A. Never fail a student with a disability
    B. Evaluate the student using the same criteria as for other students
    C. Fail a student if the performance deficits relate directly to the disability
    D. Understand that the rights of the student supersede the rights of the patients

29. By signing the final evaluation of fieldwork experience:
    A. You are agreeing with the content of the evaluation
    B. You cannot bring legal suit against the facility
    C. You are confirming that you have read the evaluation
    D. You cannot bring legal suit against the academic program

Rules and Guidelines of the Profession

AOTA *Essentials and Guidelines of an Accredited Educational Program for the Occupational Therapy Assistant* have been in existence since 1958. The intent of the document is to present minimum standards for educating occupational therapy assistant (OTA) students. Answer the following questions based on these *Essentials*.

30. Following the completion of all academic work, all fieldwork should be completed within:
    A. 12 months
    B. 18 months
    C. 2 years
    D. As soon as possible

31. The minimum amount of time required for Level II Fieldwork is:
    A. 12 weeks of full-time fieldwork
    B. 8 weeks minimum
    C. 14 weeks
    D. 440 hours

32. Level II direct supervision of the OTA student must be performed by:
    A. An entry-level registered occupational therapist (OTR)
    B. An entry-level certified occupational therapy assistant (COTA)
    C. An OTR or a COTA with at least 1 year of experience
    D. Any qualified healthcare professional such as a nurse, social worker, etc.

33. The ratio of fieldwork educators to students should be:

    A.   1 to 1

    B.   Sufficient to provide adequate supervision and assessment to ensure that fieldwork objectives are achievable

    C.   1 to 2

    D.   Sufficient to ensure that the department is able to run smoothly

34. According to the AOTA *Guide to Fieldwork Education,* fieldwork objectives should:

    A.   Be the same for Level I and II Fieldwork

    B.   Always be written by the fieldwork educator

    C.   Describe the performance expected, the conditions under which the student is expected to perform, and the criteria for evaluating a successful performance

    D.   Always be written by the fieldwork coordinator

35. Two AOTA documents that best guide the OT practitioner in making ethical decisions are:

    A.   *Standards and Practice of Occupational Therapy* and *Principles of Occupational Therapy Ethics*

    B.   *The Occupational Therapy Code of Ethics* and *Standards and Practice of Occupational Therapy*

    C.   *Report of the Standards and Ethic Committee* and *Uniform Terminology for Occupational Therapy*

    D.   *Ethical Considerations for OT Practitioners* and *OT Week*®

Answer the following questions based on your knowledge of the AOTA's *Standards of Practice of Occupational Therapy:*

36. The term OT Practitioner means:

    A.   OTR

    B.   COTA

    C.   Both the OTR and COTA

    D.   The OTR, COTA, and OT aide

37. The person responsible for orienting the patient to OT services is:

    A.   OT practitioner

    B.   OTR

    C.   Admissions committee

    D.   COTA

38. The person responsible for documenting OT assessment results is:

    A. OT practitioner
    B. OTR
    C. COTA
    D. Both the OTR and COTA

39. The treatment plan is documented by:

    A. OT practitioner
    B. OTR
    C. COTA
    D. Both the OTR and COTA

40. The implementation of the treatment plan is carried out by the

    A. OT practitioner
    B. OTR
    C. COTA
    D. OT aide

41. The decision to discontinue OT services is made by the:

    A. OT practitioner
    B. OTR
    C. COTA
    D. Discharge planning committee

Several AOTA Documents relate to supervision of the COTA. They are the *Guide to Classification of OT Personnel* and the *Entry-Level Role Delineations of the OTR and the COTA*. Answer the following questions based on your knowledge of these documents.

42. Entry-level practice is defined:

    A. As less than 1 year of experience
    B. As 1 to 2 years of experience
    C. As long as direct supervision by an OTR is needed
    D. By your licensure board

43. Intermediate level practice is defined as:

    A. Less than 1 year of experience

B. 1 to 2 years of experience

C. As long as direct supervision by an OTR is needed

D. 3 or more years of experience

44. Advanced level practice is defined as:

A. Less than 1 year of experience

B. 1 to 2 years of experience

C. As long as direct supervision by an OTR is needed

D. 3 or more years of experience

45. Close supervision can best be defined as:

A. Direct, on-site, daily supervision during patient treatment

B. The supervisor is available by phone at all times

C. The supervisor is physically present during patient treatment

D. Direct supervision during the COTA's initial patient contact

46. General supervision can best be defined as:

A. The supervisor is available when needed

B. The supervisor is on-site but not physically present during patient treatment

C. A combination of face to face, telephone, and written correspondence within a minimum of 3 to 5 hours per week of direct contact

D. The supervisor is on-site once a month

Application of Rules and Guidelines

47. It is your first week of Fieldwork II. Your supervisor requests that you complete a functional muscle assessment. You remember reading about the test in school but you never performed it. The first thing you should do is:

A. Read your textbook and do the test

B. Tell your supervisor that this test is not appropriate for you to do

C. Request that because you have not performed this test previously, you would like to observe the supervisor doing the test.

D. Take a risk and do the test.

48. By the end of Level II Fieldwork, a student should be expected:

A. To practice at entry-level competence

B. To carry a caseload of 6 to 8 patients

C. To practice with general supervision in all practice areas

D. To carry a caseload independently

49. In the area of screening, a student completing his or her last week of Fieldwork Level II could be expected to:

A. Give a written report of facts gathered during a client interview

B. Read and analyze screening data to determine if OT is needed for a patient

C. After interviewing a patient, determine that a manual muscle test is needed

D. Combine his or her own findings with other information and report it to the OTR

50. You are a COTA working in a subacute care facility. OT has received a referral for Mrs. Allison, a 78-year-old woman diagnosed with CVA. Activities of daily living (ADL) evaluations are generally completed by the COTA for patients with this diagnosis. Your supervising OTR will not be on-site until next week. Company policy states that evaluations must occur within 3 days of referral. Your best course of action is to:

A. Complete the ADL portion of the assessment

B. Contact the OTR to arrange an earlier visit to the site

C. Send the referral back with a note of explanation

D. Change the date of referral to the day on which the OTR is on site

51. As an entry level COTA, you are assigned to Mr. Kirk following his live transplant. You have read two books and have treated two patients with liver transplants in the past. For this patient, the minimum supervision you require is:

A. Close supervision by an OTR

B. General supervision by an OTR

C. Close supervision by an intermediate level COTA

D. General supervision by an advanced level COTA

52. You are an intermediate level COTA assigned to Mr. Kirk (see question 51 above). The minimum supervision you require is:

A. Close supervision by an OTR

B. General supervision by an OTR

C. Close supervision by an intermediate level COTA

D. General supervision by an advanced level COTA

53. You are a Fieldwork Level II student assigned to complete an ADL assessment. You have observed your supervisor completing an ADL assessment and your supervisor has observed

you completing a portion of the assessment. Your supervisor now requests that you perform the next ADL assessment independently. Your best course of action is:

A. Request that you have more time to review
B. Do the assessment independently
C. Tell your supervisor that you don't feel ready
D. Request to observe and coscore while your supervisor completes at least two more ADL assessments to determine your competence

54. You are an entry level COTA employed as an activities director. The minimum supervision you require is:

A. Close supervision by an OTR
B. General supervision by an OTR and COTA
C. No supervision by an OTR or COTA
D. General supervision by the Director of Nursing

55. You are a lay health minister as part of the Parish Health Ministries program at your church. One of the parishioners, Mr. Clark, is a man post CVA 1 year. He knows you are a COTA and asks you for some exercises to help get the strength back in his hand. Your best course of action is:

A. Give Mr. Clark a handout with exercises that will strengthen his hand
B. Ask an OTR for exercises that you can give to Mr. Clark
C. Encourage Mr. Clark to talk to his physician about a referral for OT services through an appropriate agency
D. Tell Mr. Clark that you cannot ethically assist him in this situation

56. You are a lay health minister as part of the Parish Health Ministries program at your church. Because you are a COTA, the minister asks you to develop an exercise program for general overall physical conditioning that will be held at the church for interested parishioners. Your best course of action is:

A. Tell the minister that this would violate OT standards of practice
B. Tell the minister that you must have an OTR on-site to do this
C. Develop the program
D. Request a physician's referral

When a violation of ethical conduct occurs, the National Board of Certification in Occupational Therapy, Inc. (NBCOT), can apply several sanctions after investigation.

Choose the best definition of the following terms.

57. A reprimand is:
    A. A formal written disapproval kept in the individual's file
    B. A formal disapproval that is made available to the public
    C. Conditions that must be met by the individual to remain certified (i.e., counseling, education, etc.)
    D. A loss of certification for a period of time

58. Probation is:
    A. A formal written disapproval kept in the individual's file
    B. A formal disapproval that is made available to the public
    C. Conditions that must be met by the individual to remain certified (i.e., counseling, education, etc.)
    D. A loss of certification for a period of time

59. Suspension is:
    A. A formal written disapproval kept on the individual's certification record
    B. A formal disapproval that is made available to the public
    C. Conditions set by the board that must be met by the individual to remain certified (i.e., education, counseling, etc.)
    D. A loss of certification for a certain period of time

60. Revocation is:
    A. A formal written disapproval kept in the individual's certification record
    B. A formal disapproval that is made available to the public
    C. A permanent loss of certification
    D. A loss of certification for a certain period of time

61. A colleague has been billed fraudulently for OT services. The appropriate agency for you to contact first is:
    A. The licensure board
    B. AOTA
    C. NBCOT
    D. World Federation of Occupational Therapy (WFOT)

62. The NBCOT publishes a quarterly newspaper listing the names of individuals who are subject to disciplinary action. The name of the newsletter is:

   A. *The Federal Register*
   B. *The Information Exchange*
   C. *American Journal of Occupational Therapy*
   D. *Disciplinary Network*

American Occupational Therapy Association Code of Ethics

The American Occupational Therapy Association and its component members are committed to furthering people's abilities to function fully within their total environments. To this end the occupational therapist renders service to clients in all stages of health and illness, to institutions, to other professionals and colleagues, to students, and to the general public.

In furthering this commitment, the American Occupational Therapy Association has established the Occupational Therapy Code of Ethics, this code is intended to be used as a guide to promoting and maintaining the highest standards of ethical behavior.

This Code of Ethics shall apply to all occupational therapy personnel. The term *occupational therapy personnel* shall include individuals who are registered occupational therapists, certified occupational therapy assistants, and occupational therapy students. The roles of practitioner, educator, manager, researcher, and consultant are assumed.

Principle 1 (Beneficence/Autonomy)

Occupational therapy personnel shall demonstrate a concern for the welfare and dignity of the recipient of their services.

A. The individual is responsible for providing services without regard to race, creed, national origin, sex, age, handicap, disease entity, social status, financial status, or religious affiliation.

B. The individual shall inform those people served of the nature and potential outcomes of treatment and shall respect the right of potential recipients of service to refuse treatment.

C. The individual shall inform subjects involved in education or research activities of the potential outcome of those activities.

D. The individual shall include those people served in the treatment planning process.

E. The individual shall maintain goal-directed and objective relationships with all people served.

F. The individual shall protect the confidential nature of information gained from educational, practice, and investigational activities unless sharing such information could be deemed necessary to protect the well-being of a third party.

G. The individual shall take all reasonable precautions to avoid harm to the recipient of services or detriment to the recipient's property.

H. The individual shall establish fees, based on cost analysis, that are commensurate with services rendered.

Principle 2 (Competence)

Occupational therapy personnel shall actively maintain high standards of professional competence.

 A. The individual shall hold the appropriate credential for providing service.
 B. The individual shall recognize the need for competence and shall participate in continuing professional development.
 C. The individual shall function within the parameters of his or her competence and the standards of the profession.
 D. The individual shall refer clients to other service providers or consult with other service providers when additional knowledge and expertise is required.

Principle 3 (Compliance With Laws and Regulations)

Occupational therapy personnel shall comply with laws and Association policies guiding the profession of occupational therapy.

 A. The individual shall be acquainted with applicable local, state, federal, and institutional rules and Association policies and shall function accordingly.
 B. The individual shall inform employers, employees, and colleagues about those laws and policies that apply to the profession of occupational therapy.
 C. The individual shall require those whom they supervise to adhere to the Code of Ethics.
 D. The individual shall accurately record and report information.

Principle 4 (Public Information)

Occupational therapy personnel shall provide accurate information concerning occupational therapy services.

 A. The individual shall accurately represent his or her competence and training.
 B. The individual shall not use or participate in the use of any form of communication that contains a false, fraudulent, deceptive, or unfair statement or claim.

Principle 5 (Professional Relationships)

Occupational therapy personnel shall function with discretion and integrity in relations with colleagues and other professionals, and shall be concerned with the quality of their services.

 A. The individual shall report illegal, incompetent, and/or unethical practice to the appropriate authority.

B. The individual shall not disclose privileged information when participating in reviews of peers, programs, or systems.

C. The individual who employs or supervises colleagues shall provide appropriate supervision, as defined in AOTA guidelines or state laws, regulations, and institutional policies.

D. The individual shall recognize the contributions of colleagues when disseminating professional information.

Principle 6 (Professional Conduct)

Occupational therapy personnel shall not engage in any form of conduct that constitutes a conflict of interest or that adversely reflects on the profession.

Reprinted from *The American Journal of Occupational Therapy*, *48*(11), 1037-1038, American Occupational Therapy Association, Inc., 1994. Reprinted with permission.

Answer Key

Section V

Ethics and Fieldwork

1. A. The obligation to help others. **2.** A. A relationship between the practitioner and a patient whereby both are bound to the truth. **3.** A. "Above all, do no harm." **4.** A. The patient's right to participate in and decide on healthcare decisions. **5.** D. Acting in a way that other practitioners would, in a similar situation, without benefit of hindsight or foresight. **6.** C. Doing one's duty despite the outcome or consequences. **7.** B. Making decisions based on the outcomes and consequences relating to those involved as opposed to simply doing one's duty. **8.** A. The decision to shorten a therapy session despite a company mandate to provide full sessions for each patient because a patient is complaining of pain. **9.** B. The decision to visit a patient on your day off because you promised to do so. **10.** A. The decision to refuse to do minimal assist transfers with a patient who has poor sitting balance when requested by your supervisor.

11. B. Talk with the supervisor. **12.** B. Talk with Mrs. Smith about potential outcomes of therapy. **13.** B. Tell your supervisor that you must accurately represent your competence and training. **14.** C. The student has acted unethically. **15.** A. Discuss the situation with your supervisor to find out the facility's policy on this. **16.** C. You have a medical condition that may endanger the patient. **17.** B. Your primary ethical duty is to Mr. James. **18.** A. Evelyn has a right to decide and pursue her own enjoyments even if her habits are unhealthy. **19.** A. You have violated your agreement to treat Mrs. Wareham. **20.** C. Report the situation to the nurse.

21. B. Your supervisor is correct because you failed to identify that Mrs. Lidwell's motivation was the largest contributing factor to any potential recovery, and may have taken away any chance for recovery. **22.** D. Race. **23.** A. The Buckley Amendment. **24.** C. Access and disclosure of information about a student. **25.** A. The Buckley Amendment. **26.** B. Medical, psychiatric, and counseling records. **27.** A. A student with fine motor problems is permitted to dictate progress notes. **28.** B. Evaluate the student using the same criteria as for other students. **29.** C. You are confirming that you have read the evaluation. **30.** B. 18 months.

31. D. 440 hours. **32.** C. An OTR or a COTA with at least 1 year of experience. **33.** B. Sufficient to provide adequate supervision and assessment to ensure that fieldwork objectives are achievable. **34.** C. Describe the performance expected, the conditions under which the student is expected to perform, and the criteria for evaluating a successful performance. **35.** B. *The Occupational Therapy Code of Ethics* and *Standards and Practice of Occupational Therapy.* **36.** C. Both the OTR and COTA. **37.** A. OT practitioner. **38.** B. OTR. **39.** B. OTR. **40.** A. OT practitioner.

41. B. OTR. **42.** A. As less than 1 year of experience. **43.** B. 1 to 2 years of experience. **44.** D. 3 or more years of experience. **45.** A. Direct, on-site, daily supervision during patient treatment. **46.** C. A combination of face to face, telephone, and written correspondence with a minimum of 3 to 5 hours per week of direct contact. **47.** C. Request that because you have not performed this test previously, you would like to observe the supervisor doing the test. **48.** A. To practice at entry-level competence. **49.** A. Give a written report of facts gathered during a client interview. **50.** B. Contact the OTR to arrange an earlier visit to the site.

51. A. Close supervision by an OTR. **52.** A. Close supervision by an OTR. **53.** D. Request to observe and coscore while your supervisor completes at least two more ADL assessments to determine your competence. **54.** C. No supervision by an OTR or COTA. **55.** C. Encourage Mr. Clark to talk to his physician about a referral for OT services through an appropriate agency. **56.** C. Develop the program. **57.** A. A formal written disapproval kept in the individual's file. **58.** C. Conditions that must be met by the individual to remain certified (i.e., counseling, education, etc.). **59.** D. A loss of certification for a certain period of time. **60.** C. A permanent loss of certification.

61. C. NBCOT. **62.** B. *The Information Exchange.*

Bibliography

American Occupational Therapy Association. (1983). *Reference manual of the official documents of the american occupational therapy association* (Rev. ed.). Rockville, MD: American Occupational Therapy Association.

American Occupational Therapy Association. (1990). Entry-level role delineation for registered occupational therapists (OTRs) and certified occupational therapy assistants (COTAs). *American Journal of Occupational Therapy, 44,* 1091–1102.

American Occupational Therapy Association. (1990). *Executive summary on rules, regulations, and guidelines governing practice by and supervision of certified occupational therapy assistants.* Rockville, MD: American Occupational Therapy Association.

American Occupational Therapy Association. (1990). Supervision guidelines for certified occupational therapy assistants. *American Journal of Occupational Therapy, 44,* 1089–1090.

American Occupational Therapy Association. (1991). *Guide to fieldwork education* (Rev. ed.). Rockville, MD: American Occupational Therapy Association.

American Occupational Therapy Association. (1994). Occupational Therapy Code of Ethics. *The American Journal of Occupational Therapy, 48*(11), 1037–1038.

Bailey, D. M., & Schwartzberg, S. L. (1995). *Ethical and legal dilemmas in occupational therapy.* Philadelphia, PA: F. A. Davis Company.

Bush, M. A. (1989). *Study guide to accompany occupational therapy for physical dysfunction* (3rd ed.). Baltimore, MD: Williams & Wilkins.

Cary, J. R. (1978). *How to create interiors for the disabled* (1st ed.). New York, NY: Pantheon Books.

Clark, E. N. *Occupational therapy trivia.* Rockville, MD: American Occupational Therapy Association.

Certification Examination for OTA 1979 through 1981 Handbook for Candidates. New York, NY: Professional Examination Services.

Certification Examination for OTA 1982 through 1983 Handbook for Candidates, OTA Examination. New York, NY: The Psychological Corporation.

Certification Examination for OTA 1984 Handbook for Candidates, OTA Examination. Cleveland, OH: The Psychological Corporation.

Certification Examination for Occupational Therapist, Registered and COTA, Candidate Handbook 1989 through 1990. New York, NY: AOTCB Testing Office Professional Examination Service.

Certification Examination for Occupational Therapist, Registered and COTA, Candidate Handbook 1985 through 1989. AOTA Programs. Philadelphia, PA: ASI Processing Center.

Dundon, H. D. (1988). *Occupational therapy examination review* (5th ed.). Flushing, NY: Medical Publishing Company, Inc.

Early, M. B. (1987). *Mental concepts and techniques.* New York, NY: Raven Press.

Edge, R. S., & Groves, J. R. (1994). *The ethics of health care: A guide for clinical practice.* Albany, NY: Delamar Publishers Inc.

Fisher, A., Murray, E., & Bundy, A. (1991). *Sensory integration.* Philadelphia, PA: F. A. Davis.

Glantz, C., & Richman, N. (1990). *Occupational therapy: A vital link to the implementation of OBRA.* Rockville, MD: American Occupational Therapy Association.

Hale, G. (1979). *The source book for the disabled.* New York, NY: Paddington Press Ltd.

Hopkins, H. L., & Smith, H. D. (1988). *Willard and Spackman's occupational therapy* (7th ed.). Philadelphia, PA: J. B. Lippincott Company.

Hopkins, H. L., & Smith H. D. (Eds.). (1993). *Willard and Spackman's occupational therapy* (8th ed.). Philadelphia, PA: J. B. Lippincott company.

Hustled, G. L., & Husted J. H. (1995). *Ethical decision making in nursing* (2nd ed.). St. Louis, MO: Mosby-Year Book Inc.

Lamport, N. K., Coffey, M. S., & Hersch, G. I. (1989). *Activity analysis.* Thorofare, NJ: SLACK Incorporated.

Melnik, M., Saunders, R., & Saunders, H. D. (1989). *Managing back pain.* Bloomington, IN: Educational Opportunities.

Moyer, E. A. (1976). *Self assessment of current knowledge in occupational therapy.* Flushing, NY: Medical Examination Publishing Company, Inc.

Parker, V. T. (1987). *Problem solving, planning and organizational tasks.* Tucson, AZ: Communication Skill Builders.

Pedretti, L. W., & Zoltan, B. (1990). *Occupational therapy: Practice skills for physical dysfunction* (3rd ed.). Philadelphia, PA: C. V. Mosby Company.

Physicians Desk Reference (44th ed.). Montvale, NJ: Medical Economics Company, Inc.

Pratt, P. N., & Allen, A. S. (1989). *Occupational therapy for children* (2nd ed.). St. Louis, MO: C. V. Mosby Company.

Ryan, S. E. (1993). *The certified occupational therapy assistant.* Thorofare, NJ: SLACK Incorporated.

Ryan, S. E. (1993). *Practice issues in occupational therapy.* Thorofare, NJ: SLACK Incorporated.

Ryan S. E. (Ed.). (1993). *Practice issues in occupational therapy intraprofessional team building.* Thorofare, NJ: SLACK Incorporated.

Taber's cyclopedic medical dictionary (15th ed.) (1989). Philadelphia, PA: F. A. Davis Company.

Trombly, C. A. (1989). *Occupational therapy for physical dysfunction* (3rd ed.). Baltimore, MD: Williams & Wilkins.

Wilkinson, V., & Heater, S. (1979). *Therapeutic media and techniques of application.* New York, NY: Van Nostrand Reinhold Company.

Index

abduction-adduction movements, 14

acalculia, 26

acceptance, stage of, 55

acromioclavicular joint, 9

acrophobia, 68

activities of daily living, 97

addiction, 87

adduction, movements, 9

ADL. *See* activities of daily living

administration, 95-114

affect, 67

AJOT. See American Journal of Occupational Therapy

alcoholism, 66

ambivalence, 63

American Journal of Occupational Therapy, 99

American Psychiatric Association, 67

amputation, 147

anger, 55, 170

ankylosing spondylitis, 38

anterior horn cells, 42

antigravity exercises, 127, 144

antipsychotic agents, 67

arthritis

    gouty, 38

    rheumatoid, 32, 38

atrophy, 11

auditory stimuli, 74

Baltimore treatment equipment, 36

bargaining, stage of, 55

bench plane, 83

biceps brachii, 6

biceps femoris, 8

bladder management, 27

boutonniere, 45

bowl stabilizer, 134

bradykinesia, 46, 141

brain injury, traumatic, 87

Bruininks-Oseretsky Motor Developmental Scale, 118

burns, 38, 153

cancer, 87

carpal bone, 87

catatonia, 57, 166

chromosomal abnormality, 22

claustrophobia, 70

cock-up hand splint, 51

coma, 154

conduct disorder, 59

conversion reaction, 55, 65, 69, 70

daily living, activities of, 97

decubitus, prevention of, 39

delays, in developmental, 28

deltoid muscle, 14

delusion, 56, 64

denial, 33, 55, 69

depersonalization, 58

depression, 55, 57, 58, 70

depth perception, 30

devaluation, of self, 22

developmental delays, 28

diagnostic related groups, 104

DRGs. *See* diagnostic related groups

drug addiction, 87

dying, stages of, 55

dynamometer, 49

echolalia, 59

edema, 146

ethics, exam questions on, 177-200

extension, movements, 8

eyeball, oscillation of, 11

fatigue, signs of, 136

fieldwork, 177-200

fingertip pads, 27

fingertip pinch, 73

flexion, movement of, 8, 10, 27

flight of ideas, 163

Freud, Sigmund, 66

"frozen shoulder," 41

gait-training goals, 73

goal orientation, 78

goniometer, 50

gout, 38

gouty arthritis, 38

guidelines, for exam preparation, xiii-xiv

hallucinations, 56

health maintenance organization, 108

hearing aid, 125

heart attack, 87

Heberden's nodes, 52

hemiparesia, 49

hip extension, 12

HMO. *See* health maintenance organization

horn cells, anterior, 42

hydraulic life transfer, 143

hypertonicity, 40

hypotonicity, 39

imbalance, metabolic, 64

indecisiveness, as symptom, 68

influenza, 32

ischemia, 42

ischium, 12

joint protection, 144

juvenile rheumatoid arthritis, 32

kinesiology, exam questions on, 1-16

kinesthesia, 28

knee flexion, 12

latissimus dorsi, 139

life transfer, hydraulic, 143

Little's disease, 87

living, daily, activities of, 97

maladaptive behavior, 62

management, 95-114

mania, 58

MCPJ. *See* metacarpophalangeal joints

media, theory, 72-85

memory, 62, 66

metabolic imbalances, 64

metacarpophalangeal joints, 44

miter box, 84

motor cortex, 19

multiple sclerosis, 87

myectomy, 53

National Board of Certification in Occupational Therapy, Inc., 101

negativism, 64

obsessions, 163

Occupational Safety and Health Administration, 107

occupational therapy intervention

  exam questions on, 115-176

    pediatrics, 117-130

    physical dysfunction, 131-155

    psychosocial dysfunction, 156-171

olfactory stimuli, 123

opponens hand splint, 52

opposition, of thumb, 38

organic brain syndrome, 166

oscillation, of eyeball, 11

OSHA. *See* Occupational Safety and Health Administration

osteosarcoma, 53

pacemaker, implanted, 153

palmar interossei, 7

palmar tripod, 7

paranoia, 65, 69, 166

paraplegia, 25

Parkinson's disease, 87

pectoralis minor, 13

pediatrics, 19-32, 117-130

perception, 126

  of depth, 30

perfectionism, 69

peripheral vascular disease, 152

physiatrist, 87

physical agent modality, 108

physical dysfunction, 33-54, 86, 131-155

pinch gauge, 50

poliomyelitis, 149

preparation guidelines, xiii-xiv

pressure mat door, 33

projection, 68

proprioception, 28

psychopharmacology, 166

psychosis, 57

psychosocial dysfunction, 55-71, 156-171

pyrometric cone, 78

quadriplegia, 149

radial deviation, 6

radial nerve, 141

radiation, 87

radius, 6

ratchet brace, 83

reaction formation, 64

reactive depression, 57

reality orientation, 156

reality principle, 63

reality therapy, 67

rectus femoris, 9

red cross, 109

regression, 71, 160

release therapy, 57

remotivation, 156

respiratory dysfunction, 132

resting tremors, 47

rheumatoid arthritis, 38

    juvenile, 32

rocker knife, 36

Rogers, Carl, 30

schizophrenia

    catatonic type, 166

    paranoid type, 166

sciatic nerve, 10

scleroderma, 54

scooter board, 129

self-devaluation, 22

self-esteem, 162

self-expression, through speech, 23

serratur anterior, 14

shoulder, frozen, 41

shoulder-hand syndrome, 42

SOAP. *See* subjective objective assessment plan

soft tissue contractures, 151

solomon bar, 72

spatial relations, 127

speech, self-expression through, 23

spine, 11

    anterior convexity of, 22

spondylitis, ankylosing, 38

stabilizer, bowl, 134

stages of dying, 55

stereognosis, 126

sternoclavicular joint, 9

stress, 64

stupor, 44

subjective objective assessment plan, 105

suicide, 163

supination, movement of, 9

"sway-back" deformity, 20

tactile stimuli, 123

tenodesis hand splint, 40, 51

terminology, 110-111

thermal burns, 153

thrombosis, 38

thumb opposition, 38

transfer, hydraulic, 143

trapeze bar, 109

traumatic brain injury, 87

tremors, resting, 47

triceps brachii, 6

tuberculosis, 87

ulna, 6

ulnar nerve, 4, 10, 150

ultrasound, 153

ultraviolet light, 151

universal precautions, 154

vascular disease, peripheral, 152

verbalization, 29

wheelchair, 121, 138

withdrawal reflexes, 27

For your information

This book and many others on numerous different topics are available from SLACK Incorporated. For further information or a copy of our latest catalog, contact us at:

Professional Book Division
SLACK Incorporated
6900 Grove Road
Thorofare, NJ 08086 USA
Telephone: 1-609-848-1000
1-800-257-8290
Fax: 1-609-853-5991
E-mail: orders@slackinc.com
WWW: http://www.slackinc.com

We accept most major credit cards and checks or money orders in US dollars drawn on a US bank. Most orders are shipped within 72 hours.

Contact us for information on recent releases, forthcoming titles, and bestsellers. If you have a comment about this title or see a need for a new book, direct your correspondence to the Editorial Director at the above address.

If you are an instructor, we can be reached at the address listed above or on the Internet at *educomps@slackinc.com* for specific needs.

Thank you for your interest and we hope you found this work beneficial.